LIFE AND DEATH
IN INTENSIVE CARE

LIFE AND DEATH

IN INTENSIVE CARE

Joan Cassell

 Temple University Press
PHILADELPHIA

Temple University Press
1601 North Broad Street
Philadelphia PA 19122
www.temple.edu/tempress

Copyright © 2005 by Joan Cassell
All rights reserved
Published 2005
Printed in the United States of America

∞ The paper used in this publication meets the requirements of
the American National Standard for Information Sciences—Permanence
of Paper for Printed Library Materials, ANSI Z39.49-1992

Library of Congress Cataloging-in-Publication Data

Cassell, Joan, 1929–
     Life and death in intensive care / Joan Cassell.
        p.   cm.
     Includes bibliographical references and index.
     ISBN 1-59213-335-5 (cloth : alk. paper) — ISBN 1-59213-336-3 (pbk. : alk. paper)
        1. Surgical intensive care—United States.   2. Surgical intensive care—New
     Zealand.   3. Critical care medicine—United States.   4. Critical care medicine—New
     Zealand.   I. Title.
     RD
     RC49.C37   2005
     617′.919—dc22   2004055302

2 4 6 8 9 7 5 3 1

For Murray

Contents

Acknowledgments

This is the first time I have been part of a research team and I loved it! I was fortunate in my colleagues.

Timothy Buchman, M.D., Ph.D., who recruited me for the ethnographic component of the study, afforded me a wonderful combination of independence and assistance. Tim made no attempt to influence or censor my writings; although I occasionally glimpsed a trace of dismay when he read something I suspect he disapproved of, he remained heroically silent. At the same time, he acted as mentor, correcting my early attempts to write an article for a medical journal, demonstrating the most effective way to deal with referees' comments, and coming up with ways to disguise cases so that the emotional valence remained while surgical and personal details were altered. I looked forward to the mornings when Tim conducted ICU rounds: The combination of uncanny clinical acuity with what seemed like complete mastery of the literature was a pleasure to observe. (The fact that he does not suffer fools gladly could be stressful for residents but enlightening for an observer!)

I learned an enormous amount from Shawn Ray, R.N., B.S.N., C.C.R.N. Not only did she respond to my questions, explaining technical terms and interpersonal subtleties with patience and generosity, but I found it inspiring to watch her with patients and families. Shawn exemplifies the ideals and expertise of critical care nursing, and observing her in action was invaluable. After more than 25 years at the Midwest Medical Center, her knowledge is profound. She is familiar not only with the shortest routes from one place to another in the hospital maze, but also with the histories of the various personalities, conflicts, and fluctuations in policy that characterize any large institution. Shawn and Tim both knew where the bodies were buried: Shawn shared, Tim remained silent— with what I took as an implicit challenge to see how much I could discover on my own. (Naturally, Shawn was not the only person I obtained information from: Casual remarks, gossip, veiled hints, and confidences from intensivists, residents, nurses, secretaries, and medical techs were all helpful.)

I cannot adequately describe the immeasurable contributions of Murray Wax, who acted as a consultant on the project. For more than 28 years, Murray has been friend, mentor, and colleague. He read and commented on innumerable drafts of this manuscript, discussed concepts and personalities, supplied synonyms, Latin phrases, and translations, and tactfully corrected slipshod grammar and spelling. Since his tragic medical accident in December 2003, I desperately miss his help and support.

I am grateful to the National Institute of Nursing Research, who funded our project (NR05124). Without their generous support, this book would not exist.

I am also grateful to the intensivists in Texas and New Zealand who welcomed a stranger into their ICUs, and patiently answered questions, explained terms, and discussed their philosophies of care. My stay in Texas was brief, but the doctors and nurses could not have been kinder or more helpful. I was in New Zealand longer: Ten weeks is probably long enough to perceive the positive aspects, but not sufficiently long to discern what anthropologist-psychoanalyst George Devereux calls the "shadow-side" of "Kiwi" culture. I found New Zealanders incredibly kind and hospitable. (To give just one example from a complete stranger: When I got lost the first night I rented a car, and ended up in the dark, on top of a hill somewhere in Auckland, I appealed to a passing teenager, who took me back to his "Mum," who arose from the flower-bed she was weeding, said "follow me," jumped into her car, and led me to my little apartment around the corner from the Auckland hospital.)

Let me note that, following anthropological convention, I have done my best to disguise the personalities and cases I discuss.

I want to thank my editor at Temple University Press, Micah Kleit, whose patience, responsiveness, and expertise were enormously helpful. Working with him has been a pleasure.

INTRODUCTION

Moonscape: The Surgical Intensive Care Unit

The first impact is like finding oneself on the moon, or a planet, light years away from the dissatisfactions and delights of everyday life. Everything is strange, different. The landscape is unrecognizable. The rules are dissimilar. It even smells different.

felt this way when I first visited an operating room (OR) in 1983. But the strangeness wore off. I learned how to dress (in fresh scrubs, with sterile cap, mask, and booties over my sneakers), where to position myself (next to the anesthesiologist on a few stacked stools during an operation), how to move (to keep sterility and not touch and thus contaminate a surgeon who has scrubbed). Although I never became fluent, I learned enough of the language to understand the exchanges between surgeons, residents, and nurses. The strangeness was domesticated, became familiar. I was able to joke with nurses and residents: when the anthropologist can grasp jokes and make a few herself, she is beginning to learn the rules—spoken and unspoken—that motivate, guide, and constrain a foreign culture.

When I entered the intensive care unit (ICU), not only the landscape and the language were unfamiliar, although indeed they were. The place seemed "deeply weird," as I said to residents who asked what I thought of the place (a few smiled as though they recognized the sentiment). It was the patients who were profoundly disturbing; most, ap-

1

parently unconscious as the action swirled around them, poised between life, death, and something else, what one might call a "living"
or "social" death. The stories of what brought each person to the
unit were disquieting, each embodying a drama, a tragedy, an ethical
dilemma moving a social being to this liminal place, this liminal state,
betwixt and between,[1] neither here nor there, neither dead nor completely alive. How does a listener twist her brain around the situation
of a man, admitted because of an automobile accident (called in ICU
argot MVA, motor vehicle accident, later changed to MVC, motor
vehicle crash),[2] who is HIV positive with serious renal disease, previously treated by the VA (Veteran's Administration), who now refuses all future responsibility for him? How about a young man found
with crack cocaine in his blood and multiple gunshot wounds, who
had buckshot in his body from a previous incident? Or a schizophrenic
burn patient who had poured gasoline on herself and set it on fire and
who, some years earlier, had been found not guilty by reason of insan-
ity of an attempt to cut the throat of her three-year-old? Or a woman,
on the way to her mother's house to attend a birthday party for her
son, whose car was hit by a truck, killing her boyfriend and two of
her three children? Or an 85-year-old MVA (or crash) victim, who
the doctors say is "doing well," which means he can be released to
a nursing home? Is that doing well? Who decides what is a "good
result"?

Such issues did not seem to concern the doctors. They cared for
the patients with equal attentiveness, be they gunshot victims (termed
VOV, victims of violence), addicts, alcoholics, or cherished mothers,
wives, or grandmothers. Perhaps this concentration on patients' bodies, ignoring their social context, was easier because most patients
were so highly sedated that their responses were minimal: someone
might flinch when a painful stimulus was applied, or "sundown" (become confused and upset at night), but a patient's social self was rarely
in evidence, except when that person was ready to be discharged from
the unit. Although family photos, children's drawings, and get-well
cards might be displayed in the room, the patients were rarely in a
condition to observe them.

The nurses, too, looked matter of fact as they carried out their
tasks. They appeared to love their work. "It's habit-forming," said
a nurse-manager while a former nurse-manager added, "once you've
worked here it's hard to go to other places." "We're the best!" the
ICU nurses often said in a half-joking tone, but they meant it. They

were proud of themselves, their competence, the unit, the ICU team. I overheard a conversation between two nurses: "I'll do it," said one. "I'll help you," said the second, who was finishing her 12-hour stint. "You don't have to. Go home," said the first. "No, I'll help you!" insisted the second woman.

The residents, too, however confused or alienated they may have felt, seemed to know what they were doing. But, for the first month-and-a-half of research, I kept getting lost. I couldn't find the bathroom, the way out, the elevator. I was psychically as well as physically lost. All that sadness, all that sorrow. (An intensive care doctor in New Zealand labeled his ICU "the house of endless grief.") I found myself sleeping ten hours a night.

I have seen photographs of ICUs. They show the intimidating technology, the inert patients, on occasion, the nurses, technicians, doctors. But I've seen none that capture the *feel* of the unit, its extraterrestrial quality, the sensation of being detached from the everyday world in a different time-and-space warp. Naturally, illness itself alters the world of the sufferer in extreme and unpredictable fashion. Anthropologist, Susan DiGiacomo, discussing her diagnosis of and treatment for cancer, speaks of "the kingdom of the sick," noting that "the seriously ill take up residence in another country for the duration."[3] This unreality, this distance, this liminality or betwixt and betweenness is intensified in the ICU, where patients are in transition, neither vividly alive nor incontrovertibly dead, with the end state in doubt.

From the Earth to the Moon

How did I get here?

It began with surgeons, whom I have studied for more than twenty years.[4] "You're my savage tribe" I tell them. The surgeon I am now working with, who tends to push things as far as they will go, informs his surgical colleagues that they are my "primitive tribe." I am fond of surgeons—as are most anthropologists of the peoples we study—even when one misbehaves and throws a "doctor fit" (the phrase comes from the mentor of a woman surgeon I studied).

In the late 1990s, a trauma surgeon who was co-head of a surgical ICU in an academic medical center contacted me. Having read my book on women surgeons, he asked if I had a student who might be interested in studying end-of-life issues in an ICU. I told him I had no students: I do not teach; I conduct research and write books. But

I wanted to learn more, thinking that I, myself, might be interested in such research.

The surgeon and I met, liked one another, and felt we might work well together. The two of us assembled a grant proposal. I wrote the ethnographic sections and offered suggestions for editing the remainder. Among the projected results, we proposed that I write a book based on my research. After some time, our project was funded by the National Institute of Nursing Research, of the National Institutes of Health.[5]

I had two conditions for agreeing to conduct the research. First, that no one but myself had access to my fieldnotes. To maintain confidentiality, I would type them at home and send copies to a friend abroad, so that in the remote chance that I was subpoenaed, I could destroy the notes on my computer and refuse to submit any information. I had spent several years working on the ethics of social science research and knew that breaching confidentiality is one of the gravest risks to the people anthropologists study.[6] Such confidentiality is urgent in a medical situation threatened by potential lawsuits and government demands for data.[7] My second condition was that I would call it as I saw it: no one else would sign, read, or approve my work ahead of time, unless I showed it to a doctor or nurse for factual corroboration. Although I might produce joint articles with other members of the research team, *my* work, including the promised book, would be mine alone. The surgeon agreed and made a good thing of it, telling everyone in the ICU that he had no idea of what I was going to say and saw no indications of what I observed and was told.

My theory is that when conducting fieldwork, or ethnographic research, the people you are studying observe you carefully and take their time deciding whether or not you are trustworthy. Some will always keep their guard up and never trust you. Others will test you. And most, after a while, will decide you are trustworthy—if indeed you *are* trustworthy. (I am convinced that most people know when someone is deceiving them, even if they do not know that they know.)

What this meant was that I had my own research project within a project. This was a comfortable position: I could do what I wanted, in whatever fashion I felt was most productive, write articles as they occurred to me, and submit them to journals for publication. Unlike my study of general surgeons, where the surgeons were nervous about being observed and did as much as possible to frustrate my research, or my research on women surgeons, where I had to locate each woman and negotiate with her individually in order to observe her at work, the fact that the ICU research was initiated by the co-head of the surgical intensive care unit (SICU) gave me immediate entrée to the site and to the people I wanted to study. The surgeon not only initiated entrance, he shepherded the project through the hospital's Institutional Review Board. More than a year later, he located another unit in Texas for me to study, when the head of the ICU in a southwestern hospital I had planned to visit stopped answering communications (a painful but eventually obvious way of saying he had changed his mind about the permission he had given to study his unit). Finally, the surgeon arranged for me to spend ten weeks studying an ICU in New Zealand to compare their ideas and practices with American practices.

When I first met him, I did not realize how fortunate I was to work with an exceptionally intelligent man who epitomizes the American surgical "can-do" outlook. He could, did, and does do everything necessary to get a job done well. We still have some disagreements about research methods; he is an academic physician, with a Ph.D. in molecular biology, committed to "hard" scientific research. But we have come to a friendly standoff: he does things his way, despite my on occasion vociferous disapproval when it comes to our joint project; I do things my way, despite his on occasion quiet displeasure.

While conducting research, I observed and reflected on situations involving patients whom the ICU personnel—nurses, residents, or intensivists—felt had extremely poor odds of surviving their stay in the unit. The first surgical ICU I studied is "semi-closed": responsibility for patients is shared between surgeons and intensive care doctors (known as intensivists or critical care physicians).

Studying the SICU, I was struck by the extraordinary competence, morale, and commitment of the nurses. When I conducted research among general surgeons, the nurses were surely *there*, but I did not pay much attention to them. Some years later, when observing women surgeons, it became obvious that OR nurses might make a woman's life more difficult by imposing a relaxed set of behavioral standards for male, and another, harsher one, for female surgeons. But I must have implicitly accepted the traditional surgical view of nurses, confirmed by their subordinate role in the OR, as the doctors' "handmaidens." (In retrospect, this blindness was probably more my fault than that of the surgeons I studied.) In the SICU, the nurses' role was too crucial to overlook. Not only did they deliver the day-to-day hands-on care that frequently meant the difference between the survival or demise of a gravely ill patient, they cared *about* patients as well as *for* them. It was the nurses who waved at patients through the glass walls as the ICU team "rounded." It was the nurses who hugged patients, held their hands, embraced grieving family members. It was the nurses I asked when I wanted to learn a patient's family constellation or "story." My awareness of the compassion and caring of nurses was extended by observing a member of our research team in action, a former nurse-manager of the unit. While conducting research in the unit, or moving through the hospital, this woman would swing into action whenever her considerable skills were needed: she responded during codes, comforted family members, instructed nurses, and encouraged new nursing recruits. It was obvious that she, and the other nurses in the ICU, loved nursing, cherished their roles, and cared deeply about the welfare of patients and their families. Reading the work of Patricia Benner[8] and spending time with an exceptional clinical nurse coordinator in New Zealand strengthened my conviction that nurses play a crucial role in caring for, comforting, and healing patients and their families. The American intensivists focused primarily on *curing* disordered bodies; the nurses too were interested in cure, but many took a wider focus as well, on *healing* the sick person.[9]

Moral Economies

> What I mean by moral economy is a web of affect-saturated values that stand and function in well-defined relationship to one another.[10]
>
> —Daston, 1993

> When the premisses of science are held in common by the scientific community each must subscribe to them by an act of devotion. These premisses form not merely a guide to intuition, but also a guide to conscience; they are not merely indicative, but also normative. . . . A spiritual reality which stands over them and compels their allegiance.[11]
>
> —Polanyi, 1946

While conducting research, I tried to understand the alien world of the ICU. The first surgical ICU I studied is semi-closed: responsibility for patients is shared between surgeons and critical care specialists. Early on, I observed disagreement and, on occasion, conflict between surgeons and intensivists about whether or not to abandon aggressive treatment for a gravely ill patient. In such situations, surgeons invariably expressed more optimism than the intensivists.

It became apparent that the surgeons and intensivists conceptualized their relation to patients very differently. In end-of-life situations, this divergence led to miscommunication and conflict between surgeons and intensivists as well as inconsistent messages to patients' families.

The existence of these differences was confirmed when I observed an "open" ICU in Texas, where surgeons have final responsibility for their patients. My ideas became even more sharply focused when studying a closed ICU in Auckland, New Zealand, where intensivists had complete responsibility for patients, deciding whom they admitted to the unit and what should be done once that patient was accepted. Reading Margaret Lock and Lorraine Daston on moral economies[12] augmented and clarified these impressions. I decided that these differences could be fruitfully conceptualized as *moral economies*.

The differing values observed among surgeons and intensivists were expressed in action, not philosophical theorizing. The notion that the two groups subscribe to contrasting ethics is mine, as is the characterization of them as moral economies.

In her definition of moral economies, Daston continues: "This is a psychology at the level of whole cultures, or at least subcultures, one that takes root within and is shaped by quite particular historical circumstances."[10]

Lynn Payer examines cultural differences in medicine, contrasting theories of illness, medical practices, and ways of relating to patients in France, West Germany, England, and the United States. In her discussion of "culture bias in medical science," she describes American doctors' "imperative to intervene," noting that British physicians question the need for technological interventions and pay more attention than their American colleagues to the comfort and well-being of patients.[13] Attitudes toward death differ as well. Payer quotes a British physician on why hospices for the dying grew up first in Britain, not America: "To accept the idea of hospice, one must accept the fact that people die" and "in the UK we strive less officiously to keep alive."[14] My observations in the United States and New Zealand (which follows a British medical model) support Payer's contrasts between

American and British medicine. Surgeons provide the quintessential example of the aggressive American "can-do" approach; when a treatment fails, the solution is to be more aggressive. Payer attributes such differences to "national character," a concept popular among anthropologists in the 1940s and 1950s but somewhat discredited since then. In a new edition of her book, Payer regrets using this term, saying that "national culture" is sufficient.

The concept of moral economies is more specific and, at the same time, more encompassing than national culture. It supports an interpretation that includes the other major participants (family, critical care nurses) in the medical drama. *Economy* emphasizes that physicians are actors within a social system that continually requires them to decide among alternatives—each bearing risks and hopes, benefits and costs. *Moral* economy detaches from the monetary marketplace and recognizes that the benefits and costs have to do most strikingly with life and death, and the terms on which life might be conducted—from utterly comatose to active participation—the qualities of life, relationships to self and other. Daston compacts these vital considerations by the phrasing, "webs of affect-saturated values." I have extended Daston's notion of moral economies in science to cover the values that affect clinical decisions, especially those at the end of life.[15]

To discuss these differing values, I could employ various classical social scientific terms.[16] None, however, seem to quite fit the intellectual, emotional, and spiritual system of values that I characterize as a moral economy. In the end, I am more interested in identifying and understanding these differences than in complex theoretical and classificatory systems.

At this stage, a case may illuminate the distinctive, and on occasion conflicting, moral economies of surgeons and intensivists, as well as the doctors' passionate commitment to these values.[17]

Mr. Burke was a 78-year-old retired geology professor who was operated on May 7 for bowel fistulas (openings), which caused a distressingly damp and ill-smelling genital region. Until developing colon cancer five years earlier, the patient had led yearly summer field trips, composed of graduate students and junior professors, to national parks. His colon cancer was operated on, he underwent chemotherapy and radiation, and was symptom-free for two years. Since the death of his wife, ten years before, Mr. Burke had lived alone. He valued his independence and was proud that he had been able to drive himself to and from his chemotherapy sessions. After two years, however, he developed metastatic cancer in his liver and had another operation to excise it.

The following year, he developed fistulas in his radiated bowel and between his colon remnant through to his anal region, probably due to the earlier radiation treatments. This caused increasing pain, discomfort, and embarrassment, and he became homebound. What he missed most was his ability to get out of the house, drive himself to doctors' appointments, and show up at the local science museum where he led Saturday morning tours. He underwent another colon resection, after which his surgeon, Dr. Gordon, told his family he had "got everything," indicating that he had removed all the cancer. But the patient then developed abscesses, which required additional surgery. Dr. Gordon had promised: "Of course, you'll be back to leading those tours," but after the two surgeries, Mr. Burke ended up with worse fistulas, now into his bladder. The wound broke down and he was now leaking urine as well.

The patient had severe sepsis (infection), which was drained in the OR, and despite the surgeon's comment that he had "got everything," the ICU staff suspected that metastatic cancer remained.

The patient's two younger sisters and his nephew were devoted to him and visited him regularly in the SICU, where he was sent after the fistulas were repaired. They told the SICU doctors that they felt Mr. Burke would "not want any of this" because a prolonged recovery would likely place him in a nursing home in a dependent living situation. They said he had been in severe pain for the last two years of his life and was miserable. What had given him joy in the past was leading his science museum tours and being able to at least drive himself to and from his own chemotherapy treatments. At a family conference, attended by his sisters, nephew, and a nurse, the intensive care physician, Dr. Mannheim, asked: "What would he have wanted?" His nephew was articulate about his uncle's wishes. He stated that everyone in the family had living wills, except for his uncle, who refused to discuss it. "They'll know what to do," Mr. Burke had told his family, although family members never determined who "they" were. The family had already contacted a funeral home to make arrangements. The intensivist told them that the final decision had to be made by Dr. Gordon, the operating surgeon.

Dr. Gordon was convinced that another procedure, to drain the fluid around his lungs, would improve help him, and, despite the doubts of the ICU staff, this was performed. The patient's condition did not improve.

At ICU rounds the day after the family conference, Dr. Mannheim decided to remove the patient from the ventilator, put him on "bi-pap"[18] and give him drugs to keep him comfortable. "His comfort is the most important thing, now" he told the residents, saying that perhaps the patient could be transferred to a private room on the floor, free of the noise and distractions of the ICU.

The intensivist saw a man whose dying was being painfully prolonged. When asked "what would he want?" family members were clear that Mr. Burke would never chose prolonged illness and dependency. When queried about the case, Mannheim e-mailed me:

> I took another look at this patient, did some calculations, did a "gut check." Numbers say, in-hospital mortality, 75% to 95%, if he gets to a nursing home, 90% one year mortality, or still in nursing home, only 10% will go home and be independent. Put the numbers together, and best case scenario is a 2% to 3% chance of making it home independent.

Mannheim was convinced that the rational, the compassionate, the medically correct action at this stage was to move the patient from "cure" to "comfort care." He noted that Mr. Burke had been seen by a pulmonary specialist whose opinion was: "never independent again, and will need indefinite period on ventilator."

Soon after the ventilator tube was removed, the surgeon made rounds in the ICU, saw the tube out, and exploded, accusing the intensivist of "trying to kill" Mr. Burke.

The ventilator tube was reinserted. The surgeon called a family conference, where (according to the intensivist) he did all the talking. This was attended by several cousins, in addition to the sisters and nephew. According to the intensivist's report, the surgeon said: "You don't want him to die, do you? All we have to do is just let him get better and he'll be okay." The family assented.

(Let me note that the intensivist and the surgeon posed two *different* questions to family members. Asking "what would he want" is quite different from inquiring "You don't want him to die, do you?")

Attempting to interview Dr. Gordon to get his take on the case, I contacted a colleague of his who warned me to stay out of it, explaining that the situation was just too hot for me to intrude. Surgeons had experienced similar problems with intensivists in the past, he said, and

I gathered that the surgeon was contemplating a formal accusation of euthanasia, a serious charge that would have momentous repercussions. "This is something you don't want to walk into," he warned, "you'd be forced to take sides."

Through another surgical colleague, I did manage to talk with Dr. Gordon, an intelligent, caring physician with a sterling reputation. We talked near the OR, where a patient of his was being prepped for an operation. Dr. Gordon was guarded. After explaining what I did to keep confidentiality, I said I understood that there had been a lot of misunderstanding and disagreement about Mr. Burke and I wanted to know how he saw what happened. He relaxed and started talking.

It was extraordinary! The intensivist and the surgeon could have been describing two completely different cases. Dr. Gordon told how Mr. Burke had been in the hospital almost seven weeks, and how he had operated and corrected his fistulas. But his abdomen kept filling with fluid (there is a duct in back that kept filling the abdomen with fluid). His abdomen was distended. They "tapped" him,[19] but then when he ate, the fluid turned white. So they started feeding him intravenously. These sorts of difficulties typically stop after conservative therapy. But the fluid got infected, he was septic, and ended up in the ICU. On Tuesday, Dr. Gordon had drained him in the OR and told the family he had done everything he could. The family figured out from this that he had said that there was nothing else that could be done for him, that he did not know what else to do. But on Wednesday, the drainage stopped. The infection was gone. The only trouble the patient had was in breathing. He had huge pleural effusions.[20] They had drained the patient's lungs before, which had been successful, and he knew draining his lungs again would work. But the intensivist refused. Dr. Gordon wanted him tapped and, in fact, when he finally was, his oxygen requirements went from 100 to 40. He knew that this was "just a dip in the road," and that Mr. Burke would recover. He was "a completely viable person." Everything was going well. His oxygen requirements were lower after he had made them tap Mr. Burke on Thursday.

Friday was Memorial Day. On Saturday, he came by the ICU and found him extubated (the ventilator tube had been removed). After sedation, said the surgeon, you need 24 hours to come back. Mannheim, the intensivist, knew this, as he had been doing this for twenty years. And he removed the ventilator tube after only six hours off the medications used to sedate him for the procedure. The intensivist talked to the family on Thursday; he swears he did not paint a dark picture; he swears the family wanted the patient off the "vent." A nurse who had been present at the family conference talked to Dr. Gordon and attempted to back Mannheim up. It seemed clear that the surgeon doubted the nurse's account. (When I questioned the nurse, she reported that the patient's nephew had inquired, "Why keep going if we know he is going to die?" The family had given the nurse the name of a funeral home in case he passed away when a family member was not present.)

Mannheim had taken the patient off the vent without consulting the surgeon. He did not call Dr. Gordon or his resident; he said nothing. Gordon never knew. The intensivist said that the family wanted him off. The surgeon contacted the family and said, "What are you doing!" and they responded that, well, Mannheim had painted such a dreary picture.

They put the patient back on the ventilator and "everything's working," said the surgeon, listing all the physiological systems that were working. "This happens to our patients on a regular basis," reported the surgeon. "Everyone thinks Mannheim is out to do physician-assisted euthanasia." The patient could not be fully awake six hours after the medications given to him to sedate him for the procedure. He was unable to take a deep breath with the drugs still working.

I asked the surgeon what he thought the patient's prognosis was. He said that Mr. Burke had a 50 percent chance of living three years out of the hospital. The patient wanted his fistulas fixed; he had talked with the patient and asked: "Are you sure you want to go through this?" and he had responded, "yes."

The intensivist sees his patients for two or three weeks, said the surgeon. He does not see them walk into his office the way they do with him, Alex Gordon, saying "thank you!" "We treat the sickest of the sick," declared Dr. Gordon, "and they get better. Mannheim doesn't see his patients afterwards, he doesn't have that experience."

When Dr. Gordon talked about Mr. Burke, he told how his nephew calls him by a nickname; I think it was "Tip." When he mentioned the nephew, he said he lives four hours away. Dr. Gordon mentioned more *personal* details about Mr. Burke than did the intensivist: he saw him awake and interacting with his family; when Dr. Mannheim met the patient, he was gravely ill, perhaps dying. I wondered whether Mr. Burke was more of a *person* to the surgeon and a *case* to the intensivist. It is, of course, more difficult for an intensivist to perceive patients as persons (although as I noted in my fieldnotes, the ICU nurses do it, as do the intensivists I studied in New Zealand).

"This really bothered me," said the surgeon. "I lost sleep for four days." Some of the intensive care doctors call us and discuss what they want to do. Sometimes they are right, he said, and he finally agrees. This time, he did not get that phone call. He never got a chance to discuss the options. It was just by luck, after performing an operation that Saturday, that he happened to stop by the ICU and saw Mr. Burke extubated[21] and put him back on the ventilator. He would have been gone in an hour.

He said he hoped if I wrote about it, it might help other cases.

What happened to Mr. Burke after he left the ICU? He remained on the surgery ward for another month and a half. His wound did not heal, requiring extensive care with a "wound vac" system, a device applied to the wound surface to suction and clean the wound. On September 1, the patient died.

Does this mean that Dr. Mannheim, the intensivist, was correct and Dr. Gordon, wrong? Not really.

We are dealing with utterly incompatible views of medical reality. To each doctor, the other's viewpoint and behavior appears not only misguided but *immoral.*

I presented this case to illustrate why such "webs of affect-saturated values" are best described as moral economies. It exhibits the "act of devotion" (it is no accident that Polanyi employs a religious allusion) with which a community subscribes to such values.[11]

The following chapters outline distinctive moral economies: the nurses' ethic of caring, the covenantal ethic of surgeons, the intensivists' ethic of scarce resources. Although I employ the term *ethic* and discuss differing *values,* the concept of moral economy is more encompassing, referring to a system of values. These values are shared; they are "held in common" by a community, a profession, a nation. Moreover, as Daston and Polanyi note, they are subscribed to by a nonrational act of devotion: they possess an emotional and, indeed, spiritual valence.[10,11]

In the American surgeons' moral economy, death is the supreme enemy to be battled at any cost. The intensivists, on the other hand, think in terms of distributing a limited resource among members of a community. Moreover, not death but *suffering* is the supreme enemy; consequently, rather than attempting to sustain life to the bitter end, intensivists consider survivors' potential quality of life.

Patients' families have their own webs of affect-saturated values that influence their trust in, or distrust of, the doctors as well as the choices they make (or refuse to make). Ethnic differences exist; these will be touched on as we examine life, death, and crucial decisions in the three intensive care units.

Hospitals, too, can have specific systems of values, shared by patients and physicians. These moral economies may have ethnic or religious bases. Conflict may erupt when two hospitals with differing value-systems merge. Such difficulties, often attributed to individuals, may have a deeper, more systemic source.

National differences in moral economies are also observable. These provide the context in which doctors,' patients,' and families' decisions are achieved. Thus, intensivists have more freedom to make difficult end-of-life decisions in New Zealand than they do in the United States; these differences are supported by divergent methods of financing medical care, by a high value placed on consensus, by legal verdicts that support, as opposed to constrain, doctors' choices, by a relatively nonlitigious society as opposed to distrustful family members convinced that a lawsuit may be in their best interests, and by a unified health care system financed by a socialist government as opposed to a patchwork, market-driven system of health care. Physicians do not impose these linked systems of values on resisting patients, they are shared by doctors, patients, and family members.

Although the notion of moral economies is central to my argument, the first four chapters of this book concentrate more on the *actors* than on their value systems. The behavior of the nurses, residents, fellows, and attending physicians in the two American surgical ICUs I studied, has profound moral repercussions affecting life, death, suffering, and family attachment. Yet few of these medical workers would characterize themselves as moral agents. Some accept the moral responsibilities thrust on them by medical happenstance, while colleagues ignore the moral implications of their work by defining their task as caring for patients' *bodies*, leaving consideration of the *persons* inhabiting these bodies to others.

Chapter 5 addresses the diverging values of surgeons and intensivists, while Chapter 6 shows how these values play out, and on occasion conflict with the values of family members, at the end of life.

Chapters 7 and 8 investigate an entirely different culture with different systems of values. The New Zealand intensivists I studied seemed less bound than their American counterparts by the "imperative to intervene" with its technological corollary. They accepted responsibility as moral agents, attempting to make decisions that were culturally and interpersonally sensitive.

Chapter 9 examines a dissimilar linked system of values held by the midwestern hospital administrators. I am reluctant to characterize these as a moral economy; the values are surely interconnected, but the accent is more on *economy* than *moral*. The spiritual reality mentioned by Polanyi is absent; their values and decisions are pragmatic, not moral. The administrators are concerned with survival in a difficult and antagonistic milieu, where medical centers compete for paying patients while attempting to cope with an expanding and constantly changing host of regulatory directives. These regulations cut reimbursement while increasing the bureaucratic requirements constraining doctors and administrators, requirements that have little connection to delivering informed, compassionate medical care or teaching young doctors how to care for and about patients.

The final chapter of this book reflects on dying in an American ICU where varied value systems—of nurses, medical specialists, and families—often conflict, and financial exigencies, dictated by outside bureaucratic fiat, can hamper the way patients and families are dealt with.

The book illustrates how differing systems of professional, regional, and national values affect life and death in the ICU. Thus, at the end of life, the New Zealand intensivists consider suffering and quality of life rather than battling death to the bitter end; physicians are reimbursed in a manner that allows them time to talk with families, establish trust, and discuss personal and therapeutic issues; and medical care is largely financed by the government, so that unlike the United States, one group or disease (e.g., the aged or kidney disease) is not favored over another (e.g., children or diabetes). In contrast, we Americans get medical care that is consonant with our mercantile value system: we get the care we pay for and are denied the care *and the caring* we do not pay for.

1

A Caring Ethic: Nurses and the Dilemma of Powerlessness

The trained nurse has become one of the great blessings of humanity, taking a place beside the physician and the priest, and not inferior to either in her mission.

—William Osler, circa 1900

I remember the days on the floor when we gave back rubs, filled water pitchers and intermittently had time to sit down (not stand and wonder what else I am supposed to be doing) and talk with a patient. Unfortunately those days are long gone.

—Personal communication from a surgical ICU nurse, 2002

When I first started studying the Midwest SICU, I was struck by the differences between the ways the nurses and doctors related to patients.

The nurses cared *about* patients as well as *for* them. It was a nurse who waved at a conscious patient through the glass walls as he walked past the room. It was a nurse who held a patient's hand when a painful procedure was carried out. (Only once, in almost 18 months of research in this SICU was a resident observed holding a patient's hand, and that resident was an exceptional woman.) It was a nurse who sat silently during an end-of-life family conference, clasping and stroking the hand of the patient's wife. (This behavior is not recorded in the audiotape our project made of this conference, but in focus groups, when bereaved family members were asked who was in charge of the patient, 96 percent responded: "the nurse.")

The more time I spent in the unit, the more impressed I was by the nurses' morale and compassion. They were the infantry who conducted the hand-to-hand battle with disease while the officers concentrated on strategy. They cared deeply about their work and the patients, and appeared to know more about patient care than the first- and second-year residents who rotated through the unit for four-week stints.

A former nurse-manager said that historically the SICU was viewed as the hardest ICU to work in because it cared for the most challenging, critically ill. Most patients had not only undergone major surgery, but also suffered from multisystem problems. The patients were extremely sick, frequently infected (having more modes of entry for pathogens), heavy, and often unable to move because of large abdominal wounds (which meant the nurse had to shift them in the course of daily care). If you trained in the SICU, this woman said, you could work anywhere else in the hospital.

When the nurses declared "We're the best!" several comparisons were implied. They were convinced that their hospital was "the best," with a stellar reputation in the region and the country. (On daily rounds, the intensivists emphasized that the hospital received patients that other hospitals lacked the knowledge and facilities to care for, so that patients who would have died elsewhere survived in this unit. "I told you we resurrect the dead!" affirmed a nurse, discussing a patient who had survived a condition that I had been told was 98 percent fatal. The nurses knew that they had more training and technological expertise than the nurses on the floor. They were also claiming superiority to the ICU nurses in the medical and cardiac care units. (In Texas, a surgical research nurse affirmed that the nurses in the surgical ICU were different: They were more outspoken and confident than those in the medical unit.)

"We've got the teamwork!" proclaimed a nurse when I expressed admiration for their proficiency and esprit de corps. The little room adjoining the nurses' lockers, where nurses ate their lunches, displayed notices where people could sign up for various activities: golfing, a hockey game, a gathering at someone's house to play Bunko, a potluck meal, a shower for someone who just had a baby, or a bachelorette party for a newly engaged woman. Christmas brought forth "Secret

Santa," where a player drew a name for whom he or she bought a gift, which was exhibited, beautifully-wrapped, in the little room. At Halloween, the nurses joined in "haunting," where an anonymous gift of candy obliged the recipient to send candy to three others.

As the nurses sat around the table in the little room, they occasionally traded "war stories" affirming their competence, quick-wittedness, and composure under pressure. "Tell them about the time you paralyzed Grandpa," one nurse urged another. Nicole related the story: One day when everything was breaking loose at the same time, they were doing a perc trach (a percutaneous tracheotomy)[1] on one patient, and an old man, she could not remember his name—"Grandpa, we'll call him Grandpa. He was a cute little old grandfather"—had an emergency. She left the trach and ran into his room where Patty, his inexperienced nurse, was terrified. She sent Patty for medication and paralyzed the patient.[2] Miguel, the fellow, finally arrived, and the nurse told him what the problem was and what she had done. "You can sign for it," Nicole had announced, "Or I can not chart it."[3] This was greeted with roars of laughter, and Sandy, another nurse, told about the day the power failed. The hospital was switching from one generator to another, but something went wrong and the emergency generator failed, and there was no power at all in the unit for 20 minutes. "It was black, black, black," said Sandy, "no lights at all, no ventilators working." She was running from one end of the unit to the other, trying to take care of all the patients. There was one gunshot patient quietly bagging himself,[4] while she went down the line with Fentanyl[5] giving shots to patients, trying to calm them while this was all going on. Then the guy who was bagging himself "seized" [had a seizure] and they had to revive him. They did not lose anyone, but it was terrible. Sandy still finds it terrifying to think about. Her colleagues nodded sympathetically.

Experienced nurses showed green residents how best to administer medications and perform procedures and tried to allay what they perceived as a callous attitude of some young doctors toward patients and families. (Whenever I wanted to learn about a resident, I asked the nurses; they knew who was technically competent and knowledgeable and who was inept and unteachable, who was caring, and who, unfeeling. I doubt if the residents realized how closely they were observed and how exactingly they were judged.) The nurses took credit for the conscientiousness and compassion of one young intensivist who had completed his residency and critical care fellowship at this hospital. "We trained him!" they said fondly. (He understood the tender-hearted nurses, as well; when he needed a new home for the family cocker spaniel, whom his toddler kept mauling, he brought in a color photograph of the dog and announced that it would have to be destroyed unless someone adopted it. Naturally, a nurse took the dog in.) The nurses also recounted how they had helped smooth the rough edges from the unit co-director, who had been unacceptably harsh and brusque when he first arrived.

The nurses always seemed to know patients' prognoses. They hated caring for people whose surgeons insisted on "flogging" them—using technology to keep the body going when death was immanent. Some surgeons would paint rosy pictures to family members. The nurses were caught in the middle; they were unable to tell the truth, as they saw it, to the family, who might inquire about the condition of a moribund patient who, according to the surgeon, was improving. On occasion, an experienced nurse might quietly help a family member reach a surgeon who had been resolutely "unavailable" for days; the nurse would page the surgeon and then hand the phone to the wife or son. They knew which surgeons were reckless, had poor results, and refused to acknowledge dying. The nurses called one such man, Dr. Dreyer, "let-'em-expire-Dreyer."

It was difficult, if not impossible, for a nurse to oppose a physician. She might hint at her opinion or quietly offer a suggestion, but the doctor—be he or she resident, attending, or even medical student—was free to ignore these hints or suggestions. Despite their wishes and claims for professional status, nurses have been trained to obey. Comparing the training of nurses and doctors, one commentator says: "While medical training can be seen as a 'toughening up' process preparing students for the rigors of a doctor's life, nurse training is an object lesson in submission, In nurse training, *others* get tough. The nurse is taught to follow rules, to be deferential to doctors, and the importance of routine is emphasized."[6]

It would be a brave—perhaps foolhardy—nurse who would openly contradict a doctor, especially a senior attending physician. What this meant was that nurses were forced to utilize traditionally "feminine" modes of disagreement: gentle suggestions, sotto voce comments, and gossip. (Perhaps as a result, the nurses' "grapevine" was incredibly efficient, extending throughout the medical center.)

Patients' Stories and the Moral Order

One morning, an attending physician, leading rounds in the unit, declared: "I don't like to think about the story, it interferes with medical care." (The patient, who tested positive for alcohol and cocaine, had reported being shot by an unknown assailant after making several wrong turns in his car.)[7] The doctor turned to me: "Someone said the story was the most interesting part. Was that you?" It was not, but it could have been, and I told him I found the stories fascinating.

I waited until rounds were finished to inquire whether this doctor's distaste for stories applied only to patients to whom one might apply an unfavorable moral calculus. He responded, "No. Although some details are part of the medical picture, I prefer not to think about the rest." Later, I asked a critical care fellow whether she, too, preferred to ignore the patient's story. She said that she no longer thinks about the story; she tries not to since she found she was joking about certain patients outside their rooms. She said she found that sort of behavior unprofessional, so now she tries to concentrate on getting the patient better.

The nurses, on the other hand, invariably knew the patients' stories. Often they volunteered the information without being asked:

She's 70; he was her high school sweetheart; they were married for a month when the stove exploded; he burned his hands trying to rescue her, but she was burned over 40% of her body.

Her boyfriend shot her. They were having an argument: she came after him with a knife, and he got his gun loaded with exploding bullets, the kind they call a "cop killer." They found alcohol in her blood.

The day after a young man, shot and paralyzed in a tragic hunting accident, was sent to the unit, an exceptionally compassionate attending informed me that the patient had been accidentally shot by a family member. "He just found out today?" asked a nurse in surprise. The nurses learned this the day the patient arrived.

Knowing the patients' stories, which they pieced together from family members, the medical chart, and patients when they were able to communicate, was only one of the ways in which the nurses affirmed the personhood of patients.

The nurses, male and female, performed a culturally female-identified expressive role in the unit. They could describe the size, sex distribution, and ages of the patients' children, the relationship between the patient and family members who visited (and those who did not), and the emotional factors associated with that particular hospitalization.

On holidays, the nurses adorned the unit with hand-cut-out snow-flakes, pumpkins, and other appropriate decorations, and on occasion, wore Santa Claus hats or Christmas tree earrings. When the local baseball team made it to the playoffs, male and female nurses festooned the unit with crepe paper. They learned patients' birthdays and decorated their rooms. The nurses were the guardians of sentiment.

The doctors, on the other hand, assumed a culturally male-identified instrumental role. Male and female doctors concentrated on disease, dysfunction, and cure; the nurses, on care. The doctors focused on the disordered *body;* the nurses were involved with the sick *person.*

Let me note that I am not claiming that the doctors lacked compassion; some were remarkably compassionate and caring. Nor that the nurses were filled with the milk of human kindness; a few were curt and somewhat rough with patients (their co-workers explained that they were "burned out"). Nor am I contending that the nurses, like the sentimentalized versions of Florence Nightingale, circulated through the unit patting fevered brows while the doctors involved themselves with brute technology. ICU nurses must master and apply an intimidating range of technological procedures, measures, and instruments; while several of the SICU attending physicians conceptualized their task as knowing how to assess and assist the patient's "will to live."

Nevertheless, a striking difference existed in the way the doctors and nurses related to patients. Here are three examples:

The doctors were examining a 97-year-old woman and needed to listen to her chest sounds from the back. "I want you to give me a big hug," said her nurse, helping her sit up. When the doctors finished examining the patient, the nurse stroked her hand lovingly.

A nurse described an exchange with an intensivist she admires (who had informed me that she knows more about critical care than he does). The doctor was examining a highly sedated patient who kept reaching for him. She finally exploded: "Goddammit, he wants you to hold his hand!"

During rounds the ICU "team" examined a patient's wound, which was being dressed. When they left, a research nurse was the only one who thought to draw the curtain to shield the glass-fronted room from view while the patient's body was exposed. When I mentioned this behavior to her, she responded that she believes God is looking down, watching what people do. "Does He have a giant scorecard?" I teased. She smiled; obviously she felt that He does.

For a time, I associated the difference between the nurses' female-identified expressive role and the doctors' male-identified instrumental one with anthropologist Robert Redfield's distinction between the moral and technical orders.[8] The moral order covers "the binding together of humans through sentiments, morality, or conscience, that describe what is right." In contrast, the technical order refers to "the usefulness of things, based in necessity or expediency, and not founded in conceptions of the right."

This correlation between women and Redfield's moral order is not so much untrue as incomplete. In making this distinction, Redfield was contrasting small, relatively homogenous face-to-face societies with large, impersonal urban situations.[9] In our society, the sentiments and behavior ascribed to the moral order are most frequently assigned to women. It is women who are *expected* to nurture small face-to-face groupings within the larger order. Whether or not women actually differ from men is almost impossible to test. They are surely *believed* to be different, however, and such beliefs affect self-image and behavior. The moral order, as defined by Redfield, has been allocated to women: from the Victorian "angel in the house"; to the early suffragists who claimed that women if given the vote would "clean up" dirty politics; to the difference theorists such as Carol Gilligan,[10] who contend that women put their priorities into maintaining relationships and following an ethic of care, as opposed to men, who are more reliant on abstract principles.[11] Florence Nightingale's "lady with a lamp," the image of the nurse as ministering angel, fits neatly into this configuration.[12]

The association of nursing with women is statistical,[13] time-honored, and symbolic. The term "nurse" derives from the Latin, *nutrire*, as does "nurture." Both refer to suckling or nourishing, a capacity distinctively female. We speak of a "nurse" or a "male nurse" just as we describe a "surgeon" or a "woman surgeon." As sociologist Daniel Chambliss observes, nursing is a "feminine" occupation, both in number of practitioners and style of work. Consequently, beliefs, behavior, and job requirements reinforce each other so that "one cannot distinguish the effects of gender (female) from occupation (nursing)." Chambliss notes that nursing exemplifies the style of the historically feminine occupations: "an emphasis on caring for others, especially dependents; menial cleaning and housekeeping tasks; relatively low pay and prestige; and an emphasis on helping those (usually men) who are in charge rather than making substantive policy decisions themselves.[14]

A Caring Ethic

A hospital secretary related a horror story about an operation on her 76-year-old mother, a fragile woman with an extensive medical history. The knowledgeable secretary arranged for a famous surgeon, celebrated for his expertise, to perform the procedure. The procedure itself was a success, but just about every detail that could go wrong in a large impersonal medical center did go wrong: the go-ahead from the cardiologist was not received until the daughter intervened at the very last minute; the mother, who had to remain awake during the procedure, knew that someone, not the surgeon, closed her, since she saw the surgeon writing in the chart and telephoning as the incision was being closed; her incision bled so much in the recovery room that it required sutures inserted by a second-year resident (when he refused to meet her eyes the next morning during rounds, the mother speculated that he might be the person responsible for the inadequate closing); despite several inquiring phone calls, the daughter was not notified when the procedure was over; the patient was kept in the recovery room for more than three hours because of a hitch in communication between the recovery room and the observation unit (OU) the mother was slated to go to; and the following morning, the patient, who had suffered a previous heart attack, was given pork sausage for breakfast. When she asked for toast, she was told they had no toaster and it would take two hours to order it; she went without breakfast.[15] The only bright spot in the entire hospitalization was that during the procedure the nurse-anesthetist kept stroking the terrified woman's arm, which she found enormously comforting. It is this sort of gesture, or its absence, that patients remember long afterward.

When the mother's arm being caressed was mentioned to a nurse-anesthetist, who worked with the surgeon who had performed the operation, she responded: "We're different [from the physician-anesthesiologists]. We're taught caring from the first day [of nursing school]; the doctors never are [taught caring]."

Nurses mention caring as a crucial component in the satisfaction they get from their work. "Come on punkin', come on," encouraged an ICU nurse as she fondled the head of a mortally ill man of 76. To a woman whose temperature she was about to take, she announced in a caressing tone: "Temperature, baby." When I said I loved the way she called patients "punkin'" and "baby," she responded, "That's because I care, and they know I care."

"'Care' is the key term in nursing's definition of itself, and crucially defines what nurses believe is their task," says Chambliss, adding, "among nurses, the willingness to care when that is difficult is the distinguishing mark of the nurse." He defines their use of the term as encompassing face-to-face working with patients, dealing with the patient as whole person, the comparatively open-ended nature of the nurse's duties, and the personal commitment of the nurse to her work.[16]

Nursing theorists underscore caring. In a book titled *The Primacy of Caring*, Benner and Wrubel write:

> Nurses provide care for people in the midst of health, pain, loss, fear, disfigurement, death, grieving, challenge, growth, birth, and transition on an intimate front-line basis. Expert nurses call this *the privileged place of nursing*. (italics in original)[17]

Another nursing theorist, Jean Watson, has a Web site devoted to her "Science and Theory of Human Caring."

A nurse in the SICU began to write poems about the unit. I found them enormously touching, conveying the tragedy and compassion of intensive care. She gave me permission to reproduce one:

Lessons for a Nurse

A young man named Tim came into my care
Muscular disease giving him a scare
Then an ulcer bled, an operation.
Fluids, pressors, blood and ventilation.

Most of the nurses the same age as he
We felt connected to his history
He worked as a counselor at a high school
My daily worries became miniscule.

Each day he taught me about bravery
As his body healed from the surgery.
His muscles were weakened, his mind alert
Couldn't breathe or move, but felt every hurt.

His eyes spoke volumes of his daily thoughts
As I poked, prodded and many pains wrought.

Mostly I saw patience in his brown eyes
At times, tears told me he felt otherwise.

Many skills perfected caring for Tim
Starting IVs and drawing blood from him.
Turning, suctioning and weaning the vent,
Positioning, physical assessment.

More importantly, one lesson he taught
That life is great, every fight should be fought.
I learned how to touch, to joke and be there.
I learned not just to give but to truly care.[18]

The Dilemma of Caring

Caring, however, can be a double-edged sword. The association of women with the characteristics of the moral order may have a "chilling effect." Nurses' salaries are low. As Chiarella points out, they have often fallen below the average living wage. Because nursing is a labor-intensive occupation, however, even a small increase in these salaries would affect the payroll dramatically. Moral pressure, arguing that an increase in nurses' pay would affect the lives of patients, has been brought to bear so frequently that such claims have became part of nursing culture.[19] In addition, as Chiarella notes, caring is so central to notions of womanhood that to demand significant recompense for it would risk nurses being perceived as heartless by the general public.[20] As a result, nurses are customarily reluctant to form unions, or join them when invited, or to threaten job actions. They feel a *personal* responsibility for patients. An increased workload means that nurses no longer have the time to care *about* as well as for patients. When working conditions become intolerable, they vote with their feet—and leave nursing. The resulting shortage makes for even more intolerable conditions, since the remaining nurses must work harder, with no compensating increases in pay. On occasion, new employees will be paid bonuses, as will nurses who have stayed for a few years. But retention bonuses to nurses who have worked in the same hospital for a long time are a contested issue. Long-term nurses feel unappreciated when they see newcomers at less prestigious hospitals being offered $4000 to sign up, with tuition loans for nursing school being paid off. The Midwest medical center issues a little pin to nurses with a tiny precious stone; the stone becomes more valuable as the years of service increase, with a diamond representing 25 years. The nurses were neither naïve nor stupid, however, and they understood that tiny rubies, sapphires, or diamonds were far less costly than the 18 million dollars I heard administrators estimate as the cost of retention bonuses.[21]

At a meeting in the SICU, the nurses discussed salaries. They were upset that the hospital paid agency nurses—whom they employed frequently to fill in when they were short of nurses—twice the hourly wage earned by experienced nurses.[22] A male nurse said he would like to stay at this hospital, he likes the work a lot, he always wanted to work in this ICU, but he's making $13 an hour, and he's 35, and he wonders how he is going to assure his future. His wife works for an agency and earns $38 an hour working weekends; the agency has employee benefits as well. His brother-in-law works for Arthur Anderson and tells him that after a year at this hospital he could become a trainee at Arthur Anderson, starting at almost $40,000 a year, with 10 percent yearly increases—there's a five-year training program. "They know we're nurses," said another woman, who had entered the room and joined the discussion: "They know we're not going to leave our patients and they count on that. And of course, we're not." Another nurse said, "I'm not here for the money, I'm working with people who care about what they do and with doctors who are the best." She indicated that she could afford to do this because her husband has a good corporate job. The male nurse said, "I like what I do. But I have to think of my future and my family's future."

I attended two hospital-wide meetings where nurses' salaries were discussed; each featured the vice president in charge of human resources, a personable, well-spoken man whose responsibilities, it seemed to me, included "flak-catching." (The term "flak-catcher" was invented by Tom Wolfe to describe an official whose task it is to receive and defuse hostility from disaffected subordinates.)[23] At the nurse's meeting, an announcement that the new starting rate for nurses would go from $13.06 to $13.51 an hour was met with silence. After the VP said that the medical center was going to just break even this year because they were initiating new construction, a nurse raised her hand and said: "My mother was recruited to a focus group to see how they felt about the new hospital slogan [the slogan was 'We care']. Where does that money come from?" After the VP mentioned demographic problems, government reimbursement rules, and the hospital's difficulties, a SICU nurse leaned over and said quietly to me: "A lot of us feel it's just talk."

At the second meeting, of nurse-managers, the critiques were more pointed. "What have you done for nurses who have been here? We're working them to death and it's not enough money," declared one nurse-manager. A colleague told how all the assistants, the messengers, the techs, had been removed so that the nurses had to do their work as well as their own, and how it took three phone calls to get anything done. Another said: "There are a lot of nurses who have been here 17 years, 30 years, are very active and productive and who literally hold the walls up." Another agreed: "We've got to keep this dedicated staff who come in day after day, 8 hours, 16 hours." "A 30 cents an hour raise is a slap in the face," said one nurse-manager, who noted that teachers receive an annual $500 salary increase. "I could go to Saint Vincent's, get a sign-up bonus, and then come back in a year and make $5.00 an hour more," observed another. All the VP could say was, "Bear with us, we're going to try to come up with something."

I was dismayed that the medical center seemed to have money for new buildings, for an array of (what I surmised were) well-compensated vice presidents, for publicity people and focus groups to devise and publicize new catchy slogans about caring, but no money to fairly compensate the nurses whose labor supported the entire enterprise. It seemed to me that what the nurses needed were some fiery old-time union agitators to challenge a corrupt enterprise and win well-deserved raises for the nurses.[24] Reading Chambliss's ethnography,[25] and Chiarella's citation of legal and professional decisions affecting nurses,[26] however, I realized that this was not necessarily a corrupt medical center or even a corrupt American system; this institutional attitude toward nurses was deeply entrenched, historically and geographically. I also gradually realized that the administrators, whose decisions I had found so upsetting, were not inevitably corrupt, that they were following the rules of an entirely different system of values, which will be discussed in Chapter 9.

Starling's Law

A few weeks after I began research in the Midwest SICU, an administrative decision was made to give the ICU nurses responsibility for the two surgical observation units (OUs), four-patient rooms where patients who had just been operated on and needed special attention were sent. Apparently no warning was given; the nurse-director, whose official title was Patient Care Director, announced the decision when (so it was rumored) both co-directors of the SICU, as well as its nurse-manager, were out of town. This was quite possibly not accidental: the wily, tough, politically astute surgeon co-director was proud and protective of "his" nurses; had he received some warning, he might have had a chance to head off this disastrous ruling. As it is, the directors returned to a fait accompli that they were unable to reverse. There seemed to be no appeal.

The OUs were two floors below the SICU, in another wing of the hospital. Additional nurses were promised, and a new OU was projected, but the present staff, noted for its competence, efficiency, and high morale, were expected to take on these additional duties immediately. Apparently the nurses on the surgical floor had complained that the OU patients were too sick for them to care for.

There was much discussion of this new policy in the little room adjoining the nurses' lockers. Most of the nurses thought this was a terrible idea, although one indicated that the nurses on the surgical floor did lack the expertise to care for the OU patients. A small, lively, extremely competent nurse told how the surgery ward used to be wonderful. They all knocked themselves out to make sure everything was done. There were not enough nurses, but they spent extra time and did everything, even though they had fewer nurses than other wards. But finally, it was too much, and the good people left. It is not great any more. She left and came to the SICU, and she thinks the same thing is beginning to happen in the SICU as well. Good people are getting disgusted and leaving. She and I agreed that once it's ruined, it can't be put back again. Someone else told how a friend of hers had left the surgical floor, as had many others, because it was so understaffed. They then hired 22 new nurses, but 24 had quit.

A former nurse-manager said that originally, the surgical ward had been working well; everyone was pulling together. But an adjoining ward was falling apart, so they took the assistant nurse-manager from the effective ward and put her in the poorly functioning ward; then they had to take the SICU assistant nurse-manager for the surgical ward. "We used to talk about Starling's Law," she said, "If you stretch muscle fiber too far, it no longer stretches, but breaks."

Most nurses hated working in the OU (the term was used to cover both small units). One of the rooms was isolated, so that the nurse, alone with four patients, had no floor nurses close by to call for assistance if needed. New nurses could not work there because there was

no one to instruct and supervise them. Moreover, there were few necessary supplies in each room. Various systems were set in place to staff
the units, with announcements posted in the SICU bathrooms. None
worked well. For a time, nurses who put in 28 hours a month overtime
could get out of OU duty. But a nurse who never worked overtime
said this was unfair; *everyone* should have to work in the OU. Conflict
erupted. With the new responsibilities, the SICU was seriously understaffed. New nursing positions had been listed but not yet filled. Day
after day, the charge nurse[27] made phone call after phone call, coaxing,
bullying, using friendship as a kind of moral blackmail to persuade
colleagues to come in and work overtime. The more expert and committed the nurse, the more overtime she worked, and the more exhausted and "burned out" she or he became. Two assistant nurse-
managers had been appointed for the SICU; the enthusiasm and commitment that earned them the position had them spending so much
time doing overtime in the OU that they lacked the time and energy
to learn their new duties.

The unsatisfactory situation limped along with last-minute decisions and sacrifices ensuring staffing for the SICU and OU, until matters came to a head six months later. One of the two OUs was particularly difficult. The high-profile surgeon whose fiefdom it was loved
to operate, as did his residents, and it was almost impossible for a
nurse to contact surgeons, fellows, or even experienced residents to
make medical decisions. Pagers went unanswered, multiple phone
calls reached no one responsible; the surgeons, fellows, and high-level
residents were unreachable or "in the OR" when needed. A highly
experienced nurse had asked an intern, who was by default in charge
of the OU, to sedate an agitated patient who had previously assaulted
someone in the SICU. He refused, telling her—according to the story
making the rounds—"It sounds like you want that sedation for you,
not for the patient." The patient attacked the nurse and the small-
sized technician who had tried to come to her assistance. The next
day, the nurse came in to work. One injured eye was shut and her arm
was swollen. Several colleagues wept when they saw her. She was told
to go home and reported that she had nightmares for several weeks
after the incident. (The hospital "grapevine," to which all the nurses
were attuned, indicated that a few days later the patient laughingly
reported that he "beat up a nurse.")

The nurse was upset, but it never seems to have occurred to her
that she had any rights or recourse. If anything, she felt guilty: She

must have done something wrong to make this happen. My impression was that many of the nurses were country girls who were relatively unsophisticated, unlike street-wise indigent patients who threatened to sue at the drop of a hat. The hospital seems to have been aware of this and offered her very little besides an apology from the high-profile surgeon who was nominally in charge of the OU where the incident occurred. She saw a counselor, who made an appointment for three weeks later, until another former nurse-manager intervened, saying firmly that she needed a lot of counseling right then.

The SICU was in an uproar. Morale had plummeted. Nurses were threatening to leave the unit. Meetings were held, pledges made, additional nurses promised. An interim solution was put in place, whereby the problematic OU was closed, with its patients going to the SICU until construction on the new unit was completed.

The unit was still short of staff, however, and the pool of committed nurses willing to volunteer to work overtime was shrinking. When the nursing Patient Care Director was asked to authorize a special bonus for SICU nurses who agreed to work overtime, she refused. "If we do this for you, we'd have to do it for everyone else," she argued. The surgeon co-director of the unit, who acted as the nurses' advocate, took action, sending an e-mail to the SICU nurse-manager and the vice president in charge of nursing, saying he was worried about the stress level of the nurses, with charge nurses literally begging people to come in and the staff becoming exhausted. He proposed closing two SICU beds, admitting fewer patients until the staffing problems were solved. The second co-director disagreed, however; he said he perceived no stress among the nurses, who in fact did not confide in him as they did in his colleague; this man stated that closing beds was a potential "slippery slope." Two meetings were held. Although the SICU nurse-manager, a motherly, nonconfrontational woman, admitted that they were most frequently two or three nurses short every night, she did not favor closing beds. Like the second co-director, she preferred going on day-by-day, week-by-week, doing the best they could. The Patient Care Director said something about bringing in agency nurses, who cost $50 an hour. "For $40 an hour, I'd do it myself!" said one exceptionally intelligent and outspoken ICU nurse. "We wouldn't want you to be overstressed," said the Patient Care Director in what seemed to be a sanctimonious tone. The upshot was that no final decision was made, although the authorities were unable at this stage to ignore the fact that a serious problem existed.

The unit muddled on. Eventually, new nurses were interviewed, hired, and trained, and the new OU, constructed and opened. The nursing Patient Care Director was transferred to another position, having confronted and offended the powerful surgeon whose fiefdom the disorganized OU had been. But a number of SICU nurses had quit, some had transferred from the unit, others had gone on a per diem basis (they earned $30 a day instead of $24, with no benefits, and had somewhat greater control over where and when they worked). Starling's Law had once again been confirmed: The muscle fiber had been stretched too far.

The incident with the intern, who disregarded the nurse's valid concerns, highlights one of the most distressing aspects of being a nurse: the disrespect with which they are frequently treated—often, although not always, by inexperienced doctors. Says Chambliss, "If there is a single dominant theme in nurses' complaints about their work, it is the lack of respect they feel, from laypersons, from co-workers, and especially from physicians. It is nearly universally felt and resented." He notes that, "even medical students put down nurses in small ways."[28] Every nurse has anecdotes about trying to tell a doctor something he or she should listen to and refuses to hear.[29] To give just one example, a gifted SICU fellow would frequently charge into the rooms of patients who were in isolation, without gowning or gloving, despite nurses' remonstrances.[30] A high infection rate in the unit had recently been reduced by insisting on such precautions, and the nurses (and I, too, for that matter) found it upsetting that this young doctor acted as though the nurses who protested were invisible and inaudible.

The strengths and problems of the nurses in the Midwest SICU reflected those of nursing in general. They may well have had higher morale than many other nurses in the medical center, and their knowledge and technical skills were, of necessity, superior. But their subordinate position made them vulnerable to attempts to economize, to the fantasy that morale and competence can be stretched thin and spread over wider and wider areas without breaking, and to disrespect from the doctors who were unable to perform their work without them. For the SICU nurses, "we care" was more than a catchy slogan to attract "health care consumers." They really *did* care. But their caring could be used against them as a weapon to keep their wages low, and it was frequently difficult for them to care about caring.

A relatively recent collection of essays titled *The Lost Art of Caring:*

A Challenge to Health Professionals, Families, Communities, and Society, has no selections that deal directly with nursing.[31] The omission does not seem to have struck the editors, a physician and a political scientist specializing in medical issues. Perhaps they just took it for granted that nurses care. Nurses always have. But the relative powerlessness of nurses means that caring has left the decision-making arena—descending downward. Funding and staffing decisions, treatment decisions, and doctors' decisions about the end of life are not necessarily influenced by caring. Caring, then, becomes the ability to feel warmly about and speak lovingly to patients, to be sympathetic to family members, to attempt to mitigate the impersonality and unfeelingness of overworked doctors. Formulating catchy slogans about caring becomes more important than devising efficient, humane ways of treating hospitalized patients. Caring becomes—to use the pejorative term that is applied by "scientific" practitioners to denigrate caring physicians—hand-holding. Hand-holding is necessary; this is confirmed by the story of the secretary's mother, whose arm was stroked by a nurse-anesthetist during a terrifying operative procedure. It is, however, grossly insufficient.

Power is the joker in the deck, determining whether or not a group can enforce its ethic. The caring ethic has been relegated to nurses, the profession with the least power. Doctors are pressed from above to be more productive, defined in terms of how much money a physician brings in. Residents and medical students are taught by faculties whose "clinical productivity" impedes teaching, advising, and mentoring. Small wonder that in this milieu, where "institutional officials speak more often of the financial balance sheet than of service and the relief of suffering,"[32] the nurses' caring ethic can be expressed only in small hand-holding gestures by a powerless group whose "insignificance" is both symbolized and demonstrated by their low salaries.

2

The Best of Times, the Worst of Times

The Residents

A changing cadre of first- and second-year residents helped care for the patients in the Midwest SICU.[1] An occasional senior resident who wanted to learn more about critical care would "rotate" through. Residents generally spent four to six weeks on SICU rotation, arriving for 7:30 A.M. morning rounds, and leaving approximately 30 hours later, when morning rounds on the following day were completed. At this time, they passed on the patients they had been caring for—each took responsibility for several—to the next resident. With few exceptions, the residents came from surgery, anesthesiology, and emergency medicine training programs at the medical center.[2]

It was not difficult to distinguish between extraordinarily good residents and extraordinarily poor ones, or as the doctors said, "strong" versus "weak" house officers. In similar fashion, when observing operations during an earlier study, I could tell when a surgeon was technically superlative or abysmally poor. I did not know enough medicine or surgery, however, to assess the finer gradations.

Weak Residents

Poor residents were easy to identify. They did not know the answers to the questions posed by the attending doctors during rounds. The abysmal ones lacked basic knowledge and made medical decisions that horrified their seniors.

A qualitative difference existed between the residents enrolled in different training programs; as a group, anesthesiology residents appeared weak, and surgical residents were often superior.[3] Naturally, there were exceptions: a few senior anesthesiology residents were outstanding. An attending confirmed my impression, however, asking if I had noticed how much more second-year surgery residents seemed to know than did advanced residents in anesthesiology.

Two Asian anesthesiology residents, who had attended medical school and practiced medicine in their own country before coming to the United States, had far more than linguistic difficulties, although, indeed, their English was inadequate. They appeared to know little, made poor decisions, and ignored potentially lethal complications.[4] A third-year anesthesiology resident did not know enough to be able to drape a patient for a procedure that required sterility. The same woman proposed to give insulin to a patient who had almost died from a dose of insulin and had been mistakenly given a second dose the following day; the third dose well might have been fatal. Another resident was unable to report what operative procedure a patient he was caring for had undergone, information that was clearly listed on the patient's chart, which he was expected to read. When fellows and attendings attempted to instruct these two young doctors, they became recalcitrant, refusing to admit error. Perhaps the traditional American method of medical teaching, based on shaming residents by publicly demonstrating and correcting their lack of knowledge, was particularly difficult for these trainees.[5] When either of these residents presented cases during rounds, with constant corrections by fellows or attendings, their peers kept carefully neutral faces or rolled their eyes at one another. "I hate it when they roll their eyes," complained a young attending to me one day after rounds. "It wasn't you, it was Jung," I reassured him. I found it frightening to think of these two young physicians loosed upon unwary patients.

"That Isn't My Responsibility"

My first week studying the Midwest SICU, I arrived at 7:15 for morning rounds and found the nurse-manager sitting in the little room adjoining the nurses' lockers, talking with two nurses. One woman, Sunny, who had been up all night, was in tears and seemed close to hysteria. She described how a patient had been sent from the OR to die in the SICU. The patient arrived "pretty much dead": her pupils were blown, she had no corneal reflex, and she was bleeding.[6] The woman had a ruptured abdominal aortic aneurysm (AAA). She and a friend had been to a show on a riverboat, where she passed out; she was taken to a nearby Air Force base, "blew" the aneurysm there, and was transferred to the Midwest medical center. The surgeon she had been referred to, Dr. Gordon (a skilled and highly regarded vascular surgeon), had said: "We've come this far, why should we stop now?" "She was bleeding out. Didn't he understand?" asked Sunny. The surgeon ordered that the patient be given "epi" (epinephrine) and blood. He departed, leaving the nurses with no written orders and no clear plan of care. Runners were coming into the unit with more and more blood; the patient was bleeding in the bed, and finally on the floor, while more blood was being administered. Responsibility for the patient's care devolved on Omar, a fellow who was on-service that night, and Josh, a resident.

Sunny wondered what the patient's family knew about her condition and asked if they could be brought into her room from the waiting room. She felt they should be given a chance to say good-by. "That isn't my responsibility," said the resident, refusing to call the family.

When the patient's trickle of blood turned into a torrent, drenching the floor, Sunny kept asking: "Is Dr. Gordon [the surgeon] aware of what's going on?" "Yes," she was told, but she didn't see anyone calling him. They were administering "blind treatment" she said, "picking treatment out of the hat." Josh kept giving orders: more blood, more and more treatment. The patient's pressure was 68 over 30.[7] "Can I make her comfortable?" asked the nurse, who wanted to give the patient drugs for pain. But no drugs had been ordered. The fellow had disappeared and the resident left the patient's room and went to bed.

Finally, Sunny asked another nurse to go to the waiting room and get the family, a task the resident should have carried out. The husband kept saying, "I don't know what to do. I don't know what to do." Sunny sent for the chaplain, but she was busy elsewhere. The patient, who arrived in the unit at midnight, was dead at 4:00 A.M. The nurse took the responsibility of talking to the family and telling the husband that his wife had died. The husband kept reproaching himself: "I should have come earlier." Sunny kept assuring him: "There's nothing you could have done."

It was necessary for a doctor to "call" it (to certify that the patient was dead). Omar, the fellow, refused: "It's not my patient. It's the resident's responsibility." But the resident had gone to bed. The nurse finally telephoned the intensivist, who came in and pronounced the woman dead.

Later, according to Sunny's version of events, the resident told her: "You did a wonderful job!" and she responded: "You sucked ass!"[8]

The next morning, the intensivist scheduled a residents' meeting to discuss the case. He told the group that he and the surgeon had been in frequent communication throughout the night, and their treatment plans had been communicated to the fellow (an extraordinarily poor doctor, who departed with no notice the following month, leaving the SICU with two instead of three fellows). The intensivist said the only thing that comforted him in this disturbing incident was that no matter what treatment they would have administered, there was no way the patient could have survived. "It's the resident's responsibility to declare the patient dead; he is legally required to ask for an autopsy," asserted the intensivist, adding, "the resident should be there when the patient dies." Throughout this discussion, Josh sat in the rear of the room with his eyes closed, looking as though he were asleep. I wondered if sleeping was his way of removing himself from a situation he could not cope with, as he did with the dying patient.

Later, the intensivist told me that he had been forced to inform Josh that he had received more complaints about him during his first two days in the unit than he had about any other resident during their entire SICU rotation. I learned that, before enrolling in the anesthesiology program at the Midwest medical center, Josh had spent two years as a surgery resident. "It wasn't for me," he said. (I wondered: did he reject surgery or did surgery reject him?) Two years later, when I inquired, I learned that Josh and the two inadequate Asian residents were still in the anesthesiology training program.

Strong Residents

Strong residents were as conspicuous as weak ones: They radiated an aura of commitment and control. These young doctors arrived early and left late; they often knew everything about all the patients, not just the ones who had been assigned to them. During rounds they knew the answers to questions posed by attendings and could cite the relevant statistics and medical journal articles. Presenting a case, they were able to filter significant information from less important data, comment on appropriate medications, and suggest "treatment plans." (Poor residents would drone on and on, giving equal weight to every excruciating detail and look blankly at the attending when asked what drugs should be administered or what physiological signs should be attended to.) One surgical intern seemed so at home in the SICU that I finally asked whether her father was a surgeon. No, a radiologist—at this hospital. Another resident reported that his grandfather had been a surgeon and his grandmother an internist in India, while his father, who had trained as a veterinarian, taught physiology at a state college. A nurse told me she was never happy when some of the residents cared for her patients; she named no names, but clearly found some inadequate; she said she was always happy, however, when Vikram, the Indian resident, was on. This was high praise because the nurses knew everything about the residents. The top residents seemed to have more endurance than their peers; after being awake all night, they showed few visible signs of fatigue and still looked and acted enthusiastic about caring for patients.

Evidence-Based Medicine

Numbers are particularly good friends to novices if they have specific rules for how to interpret them. One novice medical student wanted to look at a patient's laboratory report in order to determine whether his patient had a heart attack or not (he was instructed by his preceptor to look instead at the patient.[9]

Impersonality and impartiality are cultivated by quantifiers as much for moral as for functional reasons. It is proverbial that both require dutiful self-abnegation so as to repress individuality and interest and neither accrue automatically to quantified procedures and results.[10]

A respect bordering on reverence for "evidence-based medicine" was imparted to medical students and residents at the Midwest medical center. The attendings who instructed these neophytes made it clear that practice based on "evidence" distinguishes academic physicians from nonacademic practitioners, whose behavior might be guided by unscientific hunches, sentiments, and values.[11] Strong residents were able to cite the "evidence" backing each of their contentions and decisions.

Within this moral economy, *evidence* has a very particular meaning, differing from its use in ordinary parlance (or much scientific work), becoming a narrow category composed of studies that meet specific and rigorous criteria. These studies are prospective, the data are gathered for this study rather than being analyzed after having been collected for another purpose; randomized; double-blind; of an *n* sufficiently large to render the inferences statistically plausible[12] and placebo-controlled. While not every study meets every criterion, the more criteria that are met, the more "scientific" and the more "evidential" the findings are judged to be.

The products of such studies are statistics referring to a population. Applying these statistics to an individual patient, however, poses problems, especially when the disorders are multiple, as is usually the case in an ICU. One tactic is to try for increasing certainty in the statistics while narrowing the population to whom they apply.

Lord Kelvin's Fallacy

During a presentation on end-of-life care in the Midwest SICU, a fellow cited recent cases where patients' lives had been prolonged week after week, only to terminate in death. He then cited studies of ICU expenditures, showing the escalating costs of such ultimately fatal prolongation. His solution was "an injury severity assessment tool that would accurately predict individual outcomes at an early time period in the ICU setting [in order to] help guide care." This instrument would guide intensivists by instructing when to shift from heroic care, utilizing every possible resource to prolong life, to comfort care, facilitating a pain-free death. As legitimization for this attempt to quantify an approach to dying in the ICU, he quoted Lord Kelvin, noted 19th-century physicist:

> When you can measure what you are speaking about, and express it in numbers, you know something about it; but when you cannot measure it, when you cannot express it in numbers, your knowledge is of a meagre and unsatisfactory kind: it may be the beginning of knowledge, but you have scarcely in your thoughts, advanced to the stage of science.[13]

Why did this intelligent, moral young doctor advocate this approach to death and dying? Why did he suggest that phenomena that cannot be measured are lower on an epistemological scale than those that can be expressed in numbers? As a physician, indeed as a surgeon, he has to know that clinical expertise is as crucial as are "the numbers" that residents and fellows reel off as they go from bed to bed, "rounding" in the ICU?[14] Did he take for granted that science trumps clinical expertise, caring, and moral sensibility, even when one is dealing with—or perhaps especially when one is dealing with—an emotion-drenched subject such as dying?

In the Midwest medical center, especially among young doctors-in-training, clinical expertise often appeared to be undervalued in comparison with evidence-based medicine. The stronger the resident or fellow, the more he or she seemed to venerate evidence in this narrow sense. Although medical mentors narrated lively and illustrative clinical anecdotes, describing revered teachers with formidable clinical acumen,[15] many fledgling physicians appeared to shift clinical expertise into a disvalued category. What cannot be counted thus became "meagre and unsatisfactory."

When an experienced critical-care nurse offered an opinion about the care of a patient, the same fellow discounted her view by asking for supporting citations in the medical literature. This sounds like a nasty putdown, and she may have experienced it as such, but he doubtless felt that he was preaching and practicing evidence-based medicine. Evidence trumps experience, not to mention doctors' knowledge trumping that of nurses. (In this particular case, the nurse's experience-based recommendation proved to be correct.)

At best, however, the guidance posed by evidence is probabilistic. It is clinical expertise that guides the day-to-day behavior of a skilled intensivist. Familiar with the statistics (and their limitations), as well as with other relevant studies—such familiarity being utterly necessary—the intensivist must then decide how to apply these to a specific patient with multiple disorders. This is the *art* of medicine, as opposed to the science, and medicine is an art, a craft, and a science—as well as a business.[16]

The Art of Medicine versus Bureaucratic Efficiency

Naturally, evidence-based medicine and clinical acumen are complementary and of mutual assistance. As moral economies, however, they are unregenerate rivals. Evidence-based medicine can be used to support routinization and profound simplification, in which patients become indistinguishable atoms to be dealt with according to predetermined protocols deriving from large-scale studies. Physicians then become equally undifferentiated as they "deliver" the recipes of the protocols to these indistinguishable patients. A "population" of health care providers "delivers care" to a "population" of consumers. This then supplies the medical legitimation to health maintenance organizations, who thus are justified in imposing on clinicians a set of rules and regulations so presumably established that they can be enunciated and interpreted by interchangeable medical staff.

As forecast a century ago by Max Weber, we witness the disenchantment of the healing arts and their bureaucratization.[17] The drama of clinical expertise—including the unique artistry of the charismatic physician and the stubborn individuality of the patient—are replaced by a set of rules that claim validity as "scientific medicine," now enforced by the bureaucratic purse. The bureaucratic process is efficient, but for those so enmeshed, it is an iron cage. The linguistic symbol of this process is the change in description from the *art* of medical practice to the *delivery* of medical care (suitably routinized and prepackaged).

I observed residents and fellows in the Midwest medical center emphasize evidence construed in the rigorously narrow, measurement-dependent form. There are, in fact, other crucial forms of evidence, and the fact that these cannot be expressed in numbers does not affect their significance. I also observed older, experienced doctors possessing formidable clinical expertise, themselves worrying about the reactions of colleagues if they produced research that is non-numeric and not driven by hypotheses. As one intensivist remarked, it is easy to publish hard science studies, whereas work on softer subjects is frequently rejected by prestigious medical journals. And, when dealing with problematic subjects such as emotions, many academic physicians prefer to exhibit the findings in numbers and graphs, even when the graphs measure something only tangential to the subject under study. "Evidence-based" has become a mantra rather than a guide to expert clinical care of patients.

In the Midwest medical center, high value is placed on "scientific" medicine. In the beleaguered medical enterprises of the contemporary United States, grants, publications, and reputations—of individuals and their academic centers—are hard currency.

"Apprenticeship into a science schools the neophyte into ways of feeling as well as into ways of seeing, manipulating, and understanding."[18] When medicine is valued and imparted primarily as *science*, then neophytes, in particular, take on what are perceived as objective, scientific, ways of seeing, manipulating, and understanding. Small wonder then that young doctors in academic centers may choose to focus on evidence-based medicine to the detriment of their understanding of other, equally crucial, aspects of patient care. There is much discussion these days about how to teach "caring" to young doctors.[19] When the best and brightest young doctors, those selected for prestigious academic training programs, infer that their mentors value evidence far more highly than sloppy, unscientific emotions such as compassion, then caring is not identified as an integral part of the doctor's role and persona.

The Mystique

The strong residents, especially the surgeons, shared a macho, martial mystique. They would trade war stories about the horrendous hours they had worked and the dire emergencies they had coped with. During one such discussion, a surgical intern related how he had made an agreement to cover someone and ended up "getting burned," working 60 straight hours. The other residents groaned sympathetically, but this endurance was obviously a point of pride to the narrator. Such "complaints" can be seen as a sort of muted boasting: I did it, I survived, and I took care of the patients.

When I expressed dismay about the SICU residents' 30 hours "on" 18 hours "off" schedule, the intern told me, with what sounded like a certain grim pride, that the colorectal service was worse: they had to come in at 4:30 A.M. every day, leaving at 9:00 to 11:00 P.M., with every fourth night off.[20] "Sometimes the first meal I had was dinner," he said, "at 4:30 you just don't feel like breakfast and there was often no time for lunch."

Nevertheless, when I asserted that I thought their hours were brutal and that I was not at all sure that this punishing schedule made for better doctors, two surgical residents disagreed. There's so much to learn that you need all the time you can get, they both declared; surgical knowledge is increasing so rapidly, and they have to master so many different areas, that seven years (the length of the surgical training program at the Midwest medical center) is really too short.[21] Yes, I thought to myself, and in the course of these years, worn out by this merciless schedule, the residents learn to prioritize—doing what absolutely has to be done to improve the patient's physical condition, and postponing or ignoring the human factors: Learning about the patients as individuals, talking to family members, and reflecting about the ethical issues encountered at the end of life. After all, such "soft" activities are not based on "hard" scientific evidence. We then end up with doctors who concern themselves primarily with *curing*, leaving *caring* to the nurses.

Discussing the brutal schedule with a fellow who had been on service for 72 hours, I said I thought this was inhuman. Her response was similar to the residents': "Well, we have to cram so much learning into such a short period of time"; being "the one who had the ultimate responsibility for 72 hours was a tremendous learning experience." She did remark wistfully, however, that she has no idea what's going on in the world, she does not have time to read the newspapers; all she knows is medicine. When I replied that I thought there was no necessity for these ghastly hours, that I did not think it improved medical care or compassion, she agreed that "compassion is the first thing to go." She said: "One of the problems is that there's no model for anything else. If there were a model for another way of doing things, then we could say, 'Well, this way is better.'"

Does Rigor Impart Responsibility?

In 2001, the Accreditation Council for Graduate Medical Education (ACGME) announced a cut in residents' hours. Although New York State, in response to the Libby Zion case, had instituted rules about residents' hours, these had been widely disregarded, especially by surgical training programs. Eighteen-year-old Libby Zion came to the New York Hospital ER complaining of a fever and earache; eight hours later she was dead. Her father, a writer, mounted a legal and public relations campaign, charging that her death was the result of residents who were overworked and undersupervised. Although a grand jury refused to indict the residents, it did indict the U.S. system of residency training.

The new ACGME regulations indicated that "egregious violations" would be punished by the loss of accreditation; thus, longer hours might jeopardize and possibly close a training program. A limit of 80 hours a week was set for residents, with no more than 24 hours on call (with six additional hours allowed for teaching and transferring patients to other residents). A residency program had to provide a minimum of 10 hours of rest between on-call periods.

An 80-hour week did not sound all that horrifying to me, but the senior doctors were appalled. "This is one of the worst decisions ever made," said the surgeon co-director of the SICU, declaring that "we've allowed the system to become corrupted by decisions that have nothing to do with medical care." He noted that he had worked every other night when he was a resident. Most of the physicians who objected, mentioned the long hours they had worked as residents.

With the new hours, said the unit co-director, the residents do not feel they "own" the patients. Before the SICU was forced to restrict schedules to comply with the new regulations, a resident would sign out a patient to another, and then the second resident would sign out to the first. This would provide continuity of care for patients; the same two residents would care for a patient. Now, there is no overlapping for signing out patients. And the irregularity of the revised schedule makes it difficult for an attending to know who is on call and keep track of the residents vis à vis the patients. He said that he himself feels he "owns" the SICU patients so much that he will even telephone from Japan to find out about a patient whose condition worries him. (I neglected to tell him that I had observed at least one attending who did not act as though he "owned" the patients, no matter how many rigors he had been subjected to as a resident.)

I questioned a number of experienced physicians whose opinions I respected. Almost all (with the exception of one psychiatrist) thought the cut in hours was a dangerous mistake.[22] I wondered: Was it necessary to schedule those inhuman hours for residents in order to make them feel they "owned" the patients? I asked the co-director, who said, "That's an interesting question," but rushed off to handle an emergency with no time to respond. Is fatigue an essential aspect of caring for patients? Is that how responsibility is taught? Many years ago, I was impressed by a book that discussed techniques of religious conversion, Chinese "brainwashing," and the forced elicitation of confessions from innocent people.[23] The author, a psychiatrist, contended that people's beliefs and even identities could be altered through deliberate psychological and physical pressure, that this is what occurs during many initiation ceremonies in small-scale societies, where initiates are kept sleepless, terrified, highly stressed, and in pain. This traumatic experience, it is believed, transforms the initiates from boys to men. Is fatigue and stress one way a recruit is transformed into a physician? An internist who declared that the change in schedules was an atrocious mistake, told me that the long hours have several functions; in addition to the symbolic and "brainwashing" task of transforming trainees into physicians, fatigue teaches residents that however exhausted they are, the patient comes first.

The internist said that the reduced hours make it easier for residents to duck responsibility. These days they do not want responsibility, he complained. It is a heavy weight being responsible for the patient. The same thing is happening in managed care, he contended, and in some large group practices—a patient comes in and is upset about not seeing the same doctor; the doctor does not "own" the patient.

There is no question about surgeons owning patients. The person who operated is responsible for the outcome; this is drilled into surgical residents from day one.[24] The trauma surgeons in the Texas SICU I studied were convinced that long hours and stress were crucial in teaching responsibility and commitment. I overheard two discussing the woman in charge of resident education at their medical center. "Well, she's a Ph.D.," said one, in tones of anger and disgust; he then looked at me and asked, "Sorry, are you a Ph.D.?" "Yes, but don't let it bother you," I responded. The surgeons were incensed because Alison, who is in charge of surgical education, "coddles" the residents and medical students. "Take some time for yourself, turn off your beeper, and take it easy," said one in a mocking tone. "It's those Ph.Ds on the Residency Review Committee that messed up the hours," said the other bitterly. They felt Alison was applying industry standards based on a 40-hour week to the residents. "Only surgeons and airline pilots kill people when they make mistakes," explained one. The other described what he felt was an analogous experience when he pledged a fraternity in college. At that time they were eliminating hazing, so he did not go through it; he thinks that probably his tie to the fraternity is less strong than the guys who endured the hazing. This seemed an intensely masculine point of view to me. I wondered whether the men who railed against the cut in hours—and it was mostly men I heard complaining—were not confusing correlation with causation: they worked appalling hours as residents and they feel responsible for patients, therefore the brutal hours produce the sense of responsibility.

I was intrigued to discover that in the New Zealand ICU, the residents (who are called "registrars") worked 50 to 55 hours a week.[25] So far as I could tell, it did not affect the care patients received. When I told the Auckland residents that the attendings in the United States were worried about patient coverage now that residents' hours have been cut to an 80-hour week, they said that they have a very strong "handover." The resident who is going off service spends an hour with the new on-service resident; they work together, before one leaves and the other takes over. They told me that they achieved their shorter hours by forming a registrar's organization, like a union; the organization held three "actions"—two were threats and one was an actual strike, which was painful for everyone concerned. But now there's one registrar on for a "long day" and one for a "short day," and then a different registrar on from 4:00 P.M. to midnight, and another, on all night. The ICU registrars—there were seven for a 14-bed unit—generally serve for six months, although on occasion, one will be in the unit for a full year. What this means is that the New Zealand registrars were able to learn how to care for ICU patients and put their knowledge to work in the unit, as opposed to the system followed in the Midwest and Texas units, where green residents rotated through, leaving the ICU after approximately a month. In the American ICUs, once the residents really knew what was going on and how to do things properly, they were transferred out.[26] Whenever I mentioned the American residents' schedules, and how they had been cut from 110 to 80 hours to the distress of the attendings, the New Zealand registrars would get a look of incredulity and disapproval; several commented that they did not understand how an exhausted resident could give effective patient care. So far as I could tell, the New Zealand residents were just as committed as their American opposite numbers. There were strong residents and weak ones; as in the United States, the strong ones appeared committed, the week ones, complaining.

Whose Responsibility?

The internist's complaint about residents not wanting to assume responsibility reverberated with an outlook I had noticed among many residents. They sounded, and seemed to feel, exploited. Their workload was too high, their salaries too low. I remembered my former husband's attitude toward his residency at Bellevue Hospital in the 1950s, where the residents worked 110 hours a week for $125 a month, and seemed to have a wonderful time.[27] To check, I telephoned and asked how he had felt about his residency: "I loved it!" he said. When I posed the same question to an 80-year-old surgeon, who rounded every week or two with the SICU team, he said exactly the same thing in the same tone of voice: "I loved it!"

What has changed? The best residents still seemed thrilled about learning to be doctors. But many residents seem to feel entitled to more money for less work. Surgery, where there is no question about who has the ultimate responsibility for the patient, is experiencing a decline in applicants. In 2000, over 40 training programs failed to fill all their slots. At the same time, dermatology training programs are skimming off the top-ranked medical students.[28] The term used by medical students and residents is "lifestyle." This is shorthand for shorter hours, fewer night-time emergencies, more money.

"I Want a Life"

After listening to a guest lecturer in the Midwest SICU give a highly technical presentation on sepsis—much of which went over my head—I noticed a nurse listening with a look of interest and understanding. Sally, an advanced practice nurse with an M.A. in nursing is a brilliant woman, warm, funny, and devoted to caring for patients. After the lecture, I remarked to her: "You should go to medical school, you'd make a great doc." (In retrospect, I'm ashamed of this statement; it displays an unthinking and prejudiced assumption that being a doctor is the natural goal of brilliant nurses.) Sally responded unhesitatingly: "Thank you very much, but I want a life! I want to spend time with my husband and family," she continued. "I don't need the finer things in life. Don't get me wrong, I like money and want a house, but I don't need lots of money." Sally assumes responsibility for patients and for teaching other nurses—and residents—when she is working. But she makes it clear that her personal life, and her two young children, are just as important as her work, and she shares a full-time position with another woman, who also wishes to spend time with her family.

An administrator, who has been working in hospitals for 26 years, told me that she notices a change in residents; she thinks their language used to be more possessive: They would speak of "my patients." Now the language is more impersonal and so many of them lack passion. She smiled when she said that she remembers the old days, when a resident going on service at night would be told: "You can call me. But remember, it's a sign of weakness!"

I discussed the change in residents' attitudes first by e-mail and then in person with an intensivist, who had finished his critical care training two years before. This man was closer to his residency than many of the other attendings with whom I had discussed this. He believes there is no correlation between suffering and feeling that one "owns" patients. Part of the residency is learning, he said, and you get less education if you're working 110 hours a week and are too tired to take things in. Although one of the senior attendings is convinced that today's residents are lazy and worthless, he is not sure the man is correct. There is always a "golden age" in the past, he observed. When he was a medical student, the residents used to say: "Oh, the medical students are no good, they're not the way they were in my day, today, they're worthless and weak." And when he was a junior surgical resident, they used to say "the residents are no good, they're not the way they used to be." At 80 hours, the residents will still feel brutalized and tell future residents, "You didn't have it as hard as I did, and you're not as good as we were." "Take baseball," said this baseball devotee: "They talk about the golden age of baseball but if you watch Ken Burns,[29] you see there was no golden age; they didn't make lots of money because they weren't free agents, but they wanted everything they could get. But in those days if they didn't like it they had to go back to being laborers."

Interestingly, some months later, he sounded somewhat more ambivalent about the cut in hours, noting that with the new schedule, residents do not seem to feel they own the patients in the same way they did when they cared for the same patients day after day, night after night. The residents learn more, but know less about individual patients and feel less possessive about them; this, he said, is a significant loss.

In his e-mail he noted that medicine has changed:

> Patients are sicker now and call nights are tougher. When Dr. Johnston [the 80-year-old surgeon who "loved" his residency] trained, women stayed a week in the hospital after having a vaginal delivery (now you're out in 48 hours max and they try to bribe you to leave in 24) and people stayed a week for a hernia (now you go home 1 hour post-op). Beepers didn't exist back then, you couldn't get a middle of the night CT scan or ultrasound (since neither existed), your antibiotic choice was about 2 or 3, and essentially every patient in my ICU right now who stays for more than 2 days would have been dead back then. It's true, call was every other night, but if you ask some of the "old-timers" they would tell you about listening to baseball games on the radio or bringing in their guitar on call.

Not only medicine has changed, he said, the world has also changed. Today, there is an expectation among residents and young doctors that medicine does not define you. You have other interests and you don't want to give them up. For example, he plays the guitar and composes songs. And he doesn't want to give up time with his kids, his kids are very important to him. In Dr. Johnston's day, medicine was probably his life. Dr. Johnston did not expect to spend time with his children or go to the theatre.

I realized he was right: I suspect that Dr. Johnston, like my former husband, had a wife who assumed complete responsibility for the children, the household, the family social life. Today, many young professionals like this intensivist—and indeed my son—have wives with demanding careers, and both husband and wife share responsibility for children and household. One of the prices, then, of an egalitarian marriage, may be the refusal of the husband to cede total childcare and household responsibility to his wife; consequently, he cannot focus exclusively on his profession.

"I won't give up my kids or my songs or the Yankees," said this young intensivist. "I wouldn't give up everything and be a one-facet person. These days," he asserted, "even surgery doesn't mean the end of your life."

He noted that the financial rewards have changed, as well. In the old days, doctors didn't have to worry about their 401(k)s and money for college. He loves his work and he loves his life, he said, but few surgeons and intensivists earn enough to pay for their children's college out of current income (which is what his physician father-in-law was able to do for three kids). Dermatologists still make $200,000 a year or more. But the rest of them earn far less. And when you are a resident, earning $30,000 a year or so for up to seven years, with medical school loans to repay, and you see your college roommate making three times as much, you start to wonder.

After talking with this young doctor, I realized something else had changed since my former husband and Dr. Johnston's time: the glamor and prestige attached to medicine have dimmed.[30] As a resident and fellow, my former husband had no doubts that he was going into a lofty "calling." He was training to be a doctor, the most wonderful thing he could imagine or aspire to. He and his friends felt a kind of pity for those who were not physicians.[31] His reverence for medicine was endorsed by the wider world: in the 1950s and 1960s, announcing that one was a doctor was greeted with respect and awe. When studying surgeons in the 1980s, I remember the distress with which some men described the hostility or derision they encountered when people learned they were doctors. I wondered how many of the "strong" residents I had observed came from medical families; perhaps the view of medicine as a calling, rather than a job, had been passed down to them.

Some residents today, then, see medicine as a business and not a very profitable one at that. In 2002, three residents filed a lawsuit against the National Resident Matching Program, charging restraint of trade and eliminating competition, thus fixing, depressing, standardizing, and stabilizing compensation for resident physicians. The Matching Program, instituted in 1952, set a common date on which new residents found out who is matched with a training program, and where that program is located. Medical students list their choices of residencies in order of preference, residency programs list candidates in order of preference, and then they are "matched." So far as I can tell, the idea was that by using a mathematical algorithm, with decisions announced for all programs at once, residents would not be forced to accept a second or third choice before learning whether they had been accepted at their first-choice program.[32]

One of the problems is, of course, that residents have an ambiguous status: they are both employees, doing work that might otherwise require a higher expenditure from hospitals to accomplish, and postgraduate students or apprentices learning their specialty.[33] In the early days, residents received token compensation, from nothing to $10 a month for interns, $10 to $25 a month for residents. They lived at the hospital and were given meals; although some hospitals scheduled vacations, others did not, and expected residents to make up time lost because of illness.[34] In the 1950s, the residents (like William Nolen, Dr. Johnston, the 80-year-old surgeon, and my former husband) neither earned nor expected a living wage.[35] But, as Kenneth Ludmerer points out in his magisterial work on American medical education, the around-the-clock work and around-the-clock responsibility was offset by "camaraderie among house officers, [a] metaphorical family that evolved, and the constant availability of help" with "a faculty who took a keen interest in teaching, advising, and mentoring," and a department head who "typically commanded the unswerving allegiance of his house officers."[36]

Billable Hours

Today's medical centers, hard-pressed by competition, market forces, and shrinking reimbursement from government programs and health maintenance organizations, have enthusiastically embraced business practices and personnel. Maintaining financial viability has become a paramount aim of hospital administrators who employ the moral phraseology of a societal mission to sustain health and care for patients while striving to slash costs and increase employee "productivity."

The pressures extend downward to attending physicians, who are encouraged to see more patients—the kind who generate revenue, as opposed to the indigent patients medical centers have traditionally cared for—and spend less time on nonreimbursable activities such as teaching. (Let me note that in the three ICUs I observed, almost all the intensivists seemed to take their responsibility to teach residents very seriously. Some doctors were more conscientious than others, but morning rounds were employed as occasions to teach by most if not all intensivists. In Texas, the weekly trauma Mortality and Morbidity conferences seemed aimed more at residents than attendings, being used to teach residents what to do and not to do.)

Small wonder, then, that many residents have absorbed this "ethic of billable hours" that concentrates on the bottom line. Ludmerer mentions the "hidden curriculum"—the implicit messages, the attitudes, and values that occurs by example rather than by word.[37] Harried attendings, with too little time to teach and scant time to interact with residents as individuals, may communicate a time-is-money mentality to residents. Hospital administrators, worried about the bottom line, doing their best to increase "productivity" while cutting costs, may pass on the ethic of billable hours to residents, who then, to the horror of faculty and administrators, sue to augment their own financial viability.

3

Diverse Universes
of Medical Discourse
The Fellows

The moral economies of the sites where training programs are located affect the qualities that are valued in residents and sought in critical care fellows. A star system functions in prestigious American academic centers; authorities look for brilliant candidates who have been identified as outstanding residents. Smaller, less competitive academic centers and community hospitals focus on finding and training dedicated physicians willing to serve their communities by striving to save lives. The picture is different in Auckland, New Zealand, where stars tend to hide their light in order to blend into the group, and where caring *about* patients is valued as highly as caring *for* them.

Star-Gazing in Academic Medicine

Strong residents were identified early in their careers in the Midwest medical center. "He's an outstanding resident, who has academic medicine written all over him," said an attending about a second-year surgery resident. The attendings discuss research projects with these residents and attempt to steer them into their particular specialty. Strong residents generally have high visibility. For example, Vikram, the surgery resident who knew the condition of every patient in the SICU—not only the ones he had been assigned to care for (Chapter 2)—would stand in the front of the group during rounds, parking his clipboard on the rolling table pushed from room to room, next to the clipboards of the fellow and attending physician. He always knew the answers to the questions the attendings posed and could cite the statistics, the studies, and the journals where the findings were published. ("Outstanding" residents were more likely to be men, behavior that was perceived as enterprising from a male resident might be labeled pushy from a female.)[1]

As a relatively new specialty, intensive or critical care now has its own criteria for certification.[2] To be certified as a surgical intensivist in the United States, a candidate already trained in anesthesiology or surgery must complete a year's fellowship in intensive care and then pass the critical care boards.[3] In the militaristic medical hierarchy, the fellow teaches and directs those under him—residents, medical students, and, on occasion, nurses—while reporting to and being taught by the attending physician.

Ideally, attendings hope to recruit outstanding residents for critical care fellowships. "I think he's going to be a star," is how they describe a particularly promising new recruit. A star has clinical acumen; he or she can identify what is wrong with the patient and knows what to do to treat it. Taking good care of patients is necessary but not sufficient: They must be able to learn from others and be willing to call for help when they are in over their heads.[4] Stars are familiar with the literature and can quote it chapter and verse, they pass exams with stellar marks, and are able to teach and direct residents and motivate nurses. In addition, stars are highly visible; they give off light in their particular firmament. (A star must emit light but warmth is optional.)

Unfortunately, critical care is not one of the most glamorous or sought-after specialties. Salaries—and an intensivist is salaried—are relatively modest, emergencies are continual, and on-service hours can be brutal. Consequently, SICU fellowship candidates for the Midwest medical center were selected from a relatively limited pool.

What impressed me about the fellows in the Midwest SICU was the enormous variation in ability. Three fellows had commenced their training a month before I began studying the SICU in August 2000.[5] Omar, who had attended medical school in the Mideast and graduated from an American training program in anesthesiology,[6] was appallingly poor. During my early days of research, Omar appeared even more forlorn and out of place than I felt. During rounds, he stood at the edge of the group, adding nothing to the discussion; when questioned directly, he frequently confessed that he did not know the answer. On occasion, he would drift off during rounds to make what looked like personal phone calls. "He wanders around like a lost soul," I noted in my fieldnotes; "he looks up figures on the computer, taking far more time accessing the information than the residents, then carefully copying them down. He wanders into rooms and looks at patients, but doesn't give directions." I never saw Omar teach a resident how to perform a procedure. He would drift halfway into a room when a procedure was being taught, observe from the doorway, and then wander out.[7]

After an incident with a dying patient—the resident had gone to sleep and Omar had refused to pronounce the patient dead, arguing that it was not his responsibility—an attending physician summed up Omar's skills: "He has three strikes against him; one, zero leadership skill; two, a total inability to communicate with nurses and residents; and, three, no knowledge." When he left abruptly after a few months, the unit was one fellow short; it was clear, however, that talented residents were more able and knowledgeable than Omar, and, in fact, for a month or two, an outstanding anesthesiology chief resident acted as de facto fellow.[8]

The second fellow, Siegfried, was in some ways the diametric opposite of Omar. He had a brilliant resume, had gone to medical school and trained in Germany, and worked as an anesthesiology attending for two years before deciding to study critical care. He had a job waiting for him in his Minnesota hospital when he returned. Although he came from a middle-European background, Siegfried was raised in the Near East and spoke several languages fluently. He was a brilliant doctor, in person and on paper; when he took his critical care boards, he had one of the highest scores in the country, despite the fact that he occasionally had difficulty finding the correct medical term in English. (The residents teasingly presented Siegfried with a list of his mispronunciations, which he seemed to find as amusing as they.)

Siegfried was a high-profile human being. In fact, I was surprised to learn he was *not* a surgeon, he seemed to have the somewhat egotistical self-confidence that characterizes many surgeons.[9] During rounds, he stood next to the attending, conversing with him as an equal, and on occasion disagreeing with his directions, citing statistics and studies to bolster his opinions. One young attending declared that whenever there was something he did not know, he would ask Siegfried and learn the answer. Siegfried radiated an air of control and command; it would be a rash resident who contravened his instructions.

Everyone agreed that Siegfried was a "star"—a sought-after and highly valued quality in the Midwest medical center. On the nights and weekends when he was on call, the attendings clearly knew that the unit was in good hands. During rounds, Siegfried was the one who went to the computer to read off "the numbers," or calculate various formulae to find out the patient's exact condition or what the medication dose should be. While the attending was posing theoretical teaching questions to the residents, for example, "what do you do to [achieve a particular result]?" Siegfried was donning a sterile gown and gloves and doing whatever was necessary. I noted in my field-notes: "He's knowledgeable, active, and activist. He thinks fast, then *does*."

Despite the fact that he could be charming on occasion, there was something about Siegfried I found cold and repellent. When I mentioned to an intelligent and observant nurse that I had never seen Siegfried talk to a patient, she said he did so rarely, and then he only posed questions or orders: "Open your eyes! Raise one finger!" "That's because he's an anesthesiologist," she concluded, "they don't talk to patients, or just for a minute or two before an operation." Another nurse joined in: "That's why they become anesthesiologists." I do not remember seeing him talk to patients' families. When a resident called the family members in to the room of a dying gunshot victim to see for themselves that the unit was doing everything possible, Siegfried indicated that this was unnecessary—doing everything possible was more than enough.[10]

It seemed to me that, despite the fact that he was a first-rate doctor who took excellent care of patients' *bodies*, Siegfried exhibited a sort of muted sadism, a quality that can be observed in some surgeons as well. One day, when he was leading rounds (the attending was absent) he had an exchange with a nurse about a young girl who was shot in the abdomen by her boyfriend, who had a police record. "She'll just get better to find another gang member to hook up with," observed the nurse. "Have you seen her stomach?" asked Siegfried, referring to the fact that the patient had a colostomy. "Oh they like that, doing it with someone who has a colostomy scores points!" responded the nurse, as the two of them laughed and wrinkled their noses with disgust at the idea, mentioned by one of them, of the colostomy bag being flattened between the couple. "Black medical humor" I noted in my fieldnotes, but there was something distasteful about the joking, especially in front of the residents. Another time, when the team was discussing a police officer who had been injured when driving while intoxicated, I observed that I had heard that the patient was not the nicest person in the world, and a resident responded dryly, "He wasn't exactly grateful." "He has three strikes against him," declared Siegfried: "He's a drunk, he's a cop, and he drove when he wasn't supposed to." He continued gleefully: "I put a 14-bore needle into him with no anesthesia."[11] "Oh Siegfried!" said a resident, laughingly—but possibly also horrified. "He squeaked," said Siegfried. "He squealed," corrected a resident. "He should take it like a, like a—cop," said Siegfried, "after all, they can put 41 bullets in an unarmed man."[12]

I mentioned these incidents to no one at the time and am still not sure how much the attendings or unit directors knew—or cared—about this quality in Siegfried. Siegfried was an excellent doctor and, in my opinion, an unpleasant human being. In terms of the "hidden curriculum," the teaching that occurs by example rather than by word,[13] this star performer was imparting cruelty and heartlessness to the residents along with technical expertise.

The third resident, Lydia, was a competent, compassionate surgeon who planned to subsequently practice trauma surgery. She had attended medical school after working at odd jobs to support the education of her doctor-husband, who lived several hundred miles away with their two sons. Lydia was low profile: She stood at the side of the group during rounds she rarely volunteered an opinion or citation—although when she did, her offering was always received with respect and interest—and when she directed rounds, her method of leading was as quiet as she. After one such occasion, I noted:

> It was very different from the way the men teach; there was no feeling of challenging or putting anyone on the spot, she was just finding out what Ginny [a female medical student who was "reading" patient x-rays] knew and what she needed to learn. She was soft-voiced, gentle, and knowledgeable. The interchange was more like *conversing* than *presenting* or performing. The effect upon the others was interesting: several of the female residents chimed in with questions or comments; it seemed to me that they were speaking far more than usual, usually it's the *men* who chime in. It was as though a woman leading and a woman presenting gave them permission to speak![14]

At the same time, one rather childlike female resident incessantly contradicted Lydia and refused to follow her directions, rather like a teenaged daughter rebelling against her mother. Lydia was apparently too gentle to verbally demolish this young woman, which would have been Siegfried's response to such insubordination.

Although Lydia did not exhibit the volatile high-profile surgical temperament,[15] she did display a surgeon's extraordinary endurance. The Friday after Thanksgiving, she remarked that she was tired: On Wednesday, she had driven to her home six hours away, where she had entertained her entire family for Thanksgiving; there were 29 of them. They all stayed at her home Thursday night; she bought a whole bunch of air mattresses and there were people sleeping everywhere; then, starting at midnight, she drove back and was scheduled to be on-service the following night!

So far as I could tell, Lydia was an excellent doctor. She was also an admirable human being, intelligent, hardworking, warm, compassionate. She was not a star, however; she did not give off light.

I discovered the high value placed on star quality at the Midwest medical center when musing about the future of Clark Liu, a fellow who was recruited to fill in for several months after Omar left. Trained as a surgeon, Clark had finished his SICU fellowship the previous year; he had difficulty passing his surgery boards, however, which was required before he could take the boards in critical care; consequently, he had not yet found a full-time position in critical care. Clark, who arrived in the United States from Taiwan as a teenager, appeared intelligent and knowledgeable. Although he had graduated from an American high school, college, medical school, and surgical training program, he had problems with written English, which apparently hampered his ability to take exams. Clark was an exceptionally kind, conscientious, and compassionate man. When our project conducted focus groups composed of family members of patients who had died in the SICU, one woman described how wonderful Clark had been during her son's fatal illness: He was warm and sympathetic, kept her up to date on what was going on, and hugged her when she felt upset. When a young patient died, Clark was depressed: "You've got to keep asking the question: 'what can you do better next time,'" he said in a dejected tone. (Other doctors undoubtedly feel similar sentiments, but Clark seemed to take the loss *personally*.) I observed in my fieldnotes: "If we could just mix Clark and Siegfried, one with an enormous heart and a test-taking disability, the other with *no* heart, and test-taking genius." The nurses, who were acute observers, *admired* Siegfried and *loved* Clark. The nurse-member of our research team e-mailed me a description of a meeting between Clark and the family of a dying patient:

He was very soft-spoken and compassionate in his demeanor. He stated, "She may not make it through. She had an arrest before surgery and after. The necrosis was extensive and they could not get it all. Her pupils are fixed and dilated which may mean brain injury. Once she is stable enough to travel, we'll send her to CT scan so we'll know more." Her son asked: "Is her heart still beating OK?" to which Clark replied: "Yes, her heart is OK but she's needed a lot of blood and blood pressure medicine." Her daughter stated: "In her well days, she said she did not want to live to be a vegetable; if her brain dies, she does not want to live." Clark stated: "That's real important to know." Clark then walked son and daughter over to bedside . . . he showed them what the tubes meant . . . and encouraged them to get nearer to the patient. The therapeutic use of touch and softly spoken words seemed to help ease the grief the family was experiencing.

"Patient Care During the Day, Research at Night"

Discussing Clark with the co-director of the SICU, I told him my "crazy brainstorm," that the SICU should hire Clark to carry out the patient and family interaction that one of the attendings (whom I never observed talking to family members, except once when he was almost forced to do so) sloughed off. "The problem is," said the co-director, "that people hired by the medical center have to," he hesitated. "They have to be stars," I prompted. "Yes," he agreed, "Patient care during the day, research at night." So far as I could tell, the co-director did not think I had advanced a poor idea, it was just that the system did not allow for it. What the system valued was evidence-based practice and research that produced "evidence."

SICU fellows spent time conducting basic research. Their training emphasized that a star at a prestigious medical center ICU is expected to do more than merely care for patients; he or she must also conduct scientific research that garners grants, is cited by colleagues, and promotes the national and international reputation of the institution.

Light versus Warmth

The value placed on giving off light as opposed to warmth affected relations between the SICU doctors and patients' family members. Focusing on getting the patient better is effective—when the patient improves and leaves the unit. But 9 percent of the Midwest SICU patients did not survive.[16] At such a time, *warmth* as opposed to the *light* a star emits, makes a crucial difference. Even when a patient does survive, sympathy and empathy are comforting to terrified family members who want to talk to the doctor, learn what is going on, and what the prognosis is likely to be. When the patient is dying, the doctor has little more than empathy and compassion to offer the family. And many doctors do not have these in their repertoires. The focus on star quality in academic medicine tends to select trainees like Siegfried, who may be brilliant doctors but who are not necessarily caring human beings.

In a moral economy that emphasizes brilliance and the ability to conduct hard science, the more human virtues may be short-changed. Adorning the walls with plaques bearing the slogan "We care"—does not substitute for caring behavior. The authorities at the Midwest medical center have no prejudice against compassion, it just doesn't enter into the equation when seeking and training potential stars.

Serving the Community, Saving Lives

In the Texas SICU, it seemed to be more or less taken for granted, without discussion, that a medium-sized[17] financially struggling university hospital in south Texas that was (as described to me by one doctor) as close to a community hospital as possible, was not a site that went out of its way to seek stars.

A surgical resident said that he had chosen the Texas training program because it did not schedule a year or two in the laboratory. This ruled out any possibility of academic medicine; this young doctor wanted to practice surgery and take care of patients. Although private practice is considered a step below academic medicine in the medical prestige system, many young people go into medicine to care for sick people and seek training that will prepare them for this. An aspiring star would apply to a prestigious training program at a renowned medical center, which would train him or her to shine in the medical firmament.

The Texas SICU was run by the five trauma surgeons at the medical center, one of whom acted as "fellow." The year spent as fellow allowed him to take the critical care boards that, when passed, would qualify him as an intensivist.

I did not observe the "fellow" being tutored by the other attendings. Only one of the three surgeons who concentrated on the SICU, the chief, was certified in critical care. The third man spoke of his plans to spend a subsequent year as "fellow" to also certify as an intensivist.

The fellow's office was adjacent to those of the other four trauma surgeons, two flights down from the SICU, in the same hospital wing. Unlike the fellows in the Midwest SICU, where one was usually on site, the Texas fellow spent a good deal of time in his office, fulfilling his responsibilities as trauma surgeon. In case of an emergency, one of the surgeons—not necessarily the fellow—would race up the stairs to deal with it.

In this unit, the intermediary role, filled by the Midwest SICU fellows, was taken by two third-year surgery residents who spent a month's rotation supervising and teaching medical students and less-advanced residents, and being, in turn, taught by the three trauma surgeons (one of whom was titular "fellow").

In the Texas SICU, the fellowship year seemed more of a bureaucratic necessity than an intermediate phase between resident and attending. I'm not sure how much the fellow was actually learning during this time (except for the information absorbed while preparing for his critical care boards), although qualifying as an intensivist would surely increase his prestige and salary. The fellow seemed intelligent, knowledgeable, and competent, as indeed did the trauma surgeon who had not yet completed a fellowship year. As a born and bred New Yorker, I found this trauma-surgeon-fellow exotic and opaque; although I have observed his like in films and on TV, this was the first time I had encountered a prototypical "Texan" in person. He wore cowboy boots, drove a truck—it would not have surprised me if he had a shotgun on a rack in back of his seat,[18] chewed tobacco— "dipped" was the local term for this, and claimed that he left Texas only under duress.

"A Field Filled with Oddballs"

"Critical care tends to attract oddballs," confided a New Zealand intensivist. Most of the Auckland attendings did, indeed, have unique and memorable personalities. "Edward is the only normal one," I responded, echoing Edward's recurrent plaint: "I'm the only normal one here." "Don't you believe it," declared his colleague, "he's only joking when he says that!"

A few days earlier, the intensivist had said that he would like to recruit another oddball for the ICU. As he displayed the outline of a lecture he was about to deliver to medical students, and another he gives to registrars considering what specialty to go into, I noted that one of the qualifications he had listed for critical care was that it is filled with oddballs. My interpretation of "oddball" is someone brilliant, opinionated, and interesting, if difficult, rather than a mild self-effacing solid unbrilliant intensivist, such as Greg, who was the fellow the year I was there.

Greg was so low-key that one might forget he was present when surrounded by the higher-profile attendings. This was the second fellow the unit had trained; the first, a woman, worked as an intensivist in another New Zealand ICU. Greg rotated on-call days and weekends with the six attendings. Since rounds had at least two doctors present, the on-call intensivist and the "backup," and the intensivists' offices were in the unit, an attending was almost always present to coach or correct the fellow when necessary. When an attending did instruct Greg, it was done quietly and inconspicuously; the American method of teaching by humiliation was, so far as I could tell, not employed in the Auckland ICU.

Greg seemed a devoted, careful, competent physician who was eclipsed by the more colorful attendings. He was certainly *not* an "oddball," and I got the feeling that a few attendings may have regretted this. He was, however, hardworking, reliable, conscientious, and kind. These qualities may be as essential as brilliance when caring for patients and dealing with distraught families. Like the Auckland intensivists, Greg cared about as well as for patients. He spoke to them warmly, took pains to update family members about the condition of their loved ones, and was thoughtful to residents and nurses, requesting rather than ordering and never speaking in a patronizing tone. I suspect he will become an excellent, if unmemorable intensivist.

4

The Attendings

The Star System in the Midwest Medical Center

The seven critical care doctors who cared for patients in the Midwest SICU were all stars.[1] All had passed at least two qualifying boards, one for anesthesia or surgery, and another for critical care. Several had passed three, and at least one was "boarded"—as doctors say—in four specialties.[2] One intensivist was the chief of anesthesiology; another, who held an endowed chair in the medical school, was the head of trauma surgery. All conducted research. Two of the younger attendings had been granted five-year mentored career development awards from the National Institutes of Health (NIH) in recognition not only of their research performance and potential, but also of the excellence of their mentors and the research site (the medical center). All the attendings had an impressive record of publications; some had international reputations as researchers. They were a brilliant high-powered team. This star power almost went without saying in a medical center that prided itself as much on its members' scientific accomplishments as on their ability to save lives that might have been lost in less-distinguished medical settings. The prestige system in medicine is clear: who looks down on whom. The doctors at the Midwest medical center were high in the status system, outclassed only by physicians at a few renowned university centers. These doctors outranked colleagues in less-prestigious university centers, who themselves indicated that they felt superior to private practitioners who might earn more money but, in their opinion, had less moral and social status.[3]

The *U.S. News and World Report*'s yearly rating of hospitals was eagerly awaited at the medical center, and the center's ranking, as compared with competing institutions, anxiously scrutinized. Although the rating affected patient choices, more than "merchandising" was involved. The senior administrators and the physicians seemed to take it for granted that a high ranking, like the scientific reputation of the medical center, added up to better care for patients. Surely, a greater chance at surviving whatever condition brought a patient to the hospital can be defined as "better care." However, I observed costs as well as benefits associated with the star system and the emphasis on hard science, for care has other aspects, as well.

Among the audience for the critical care fellow's presentation on quantifying dying (Chapter 2) was an ICU attending who conducts innovative scientific research as well as practicing compassionate and clinically astute medical care. When I remarked that I thought the statement of Lord Kelvin (declaring that knowledge that cannot be expressed in numbers is "meager and unsatisfactory") was nonsense, he was silent, as though nonplussed. I ventured to interpret his silence: "Oh, do you mean that as a hard scientist you agree, but as an intensivist you believe it to be nonsense?" His face cleared. Yes, that is what he meant.

Implicitly, this interplay reveals some of the complexities and contradictions inherent in the ambitions, labors, and responsibilities of those striving within the milieu of an elite academic hospital. Measurement is essential in the scientific research conducted by the attendings; what cannot be measured—love, compassion, grief, terror, sadness, and fear of death—may unthinkingly be assigned less value, even by experienced intensive care physicians who, when they reflect, are well aware of the vital importance of such human elements to patients and their families.

As well as carrying out basic or "translational" research, studying disease processes and patterns, some of the SICU attendings also conducted clinical research, testing the relative efficacy of various procedures, medications, and technologies. Scientific research offers these academic luminaries inner and outer rewards. Several mentioned the intellectual challenge and the satisfaction of unraveling a problem. Publications, awards, and grants heighten reputation—local, national, international. As the investigator's name becomes known, the work is cited by colleagues, invitations to lecture multiply, and posts at competing institutions are proffered. These rewards are more personal than the institutional rewards garnered from working in an ICU renowned for its exceptional patient care.

Serious research, however, demands time and drains emotional energy. Not merely the scientific questions, but the practical requirements are time consuming. Assistants—laboratory and other—must be located, trained, and supervised, only then perhaps to move on. Time and effort must be wagered in the lottery of grants by the crafting of applications to benevolent agencies, an unending series of investments, where each application must be formulated in accordance with the agency's particular format and project a plausible and worthy outcome. Meanwhile, letters of appraisal or recommendation must be obtained from colleagues and seniors. Since publications increase the likelihood of future funding, research reports also must be drafted, and then usually redrafted in response to the critiques of journal referees. The intensivists spent 3 to 17 weeks a year working as attendings in the SICU. The rest of the time, they were busy with other responsibilities: research, teaching, operating, acting as an administrator.

Part-Time Intensivists

The fact that the intensivists were not full time had consequences, some intended others unrecognized. Only one attending at a time was on call. This was a heavy responsibility: being in the unit or easily reachable 24 hours a day for seven days; conducting morning and afternoon rounds; teaching and directing fellows, residents, and nurses; deciding when and whether to admit new patients (which, when beds were in short supply, might involve a balancing act between several surgeons, all of whom were convinced their candidate's need for the unit was critical); determining when a patient was ready to be discharged from the ICU; updating family members about the condition of the patient; and conducting meetings with the family when a patient's condition was terminal. On occasion, if an intensivist had an urgent commitment, a colleague might substitute for him for a day or longer. But the responsibility, and decisions, belonged to the individual physician, not to the intensivists as a group.

The fact that attendings rotated every week affected patient care. Each intensivist had a distinct style of teaching and practice, related differently to patients, favored different drugs and procedures, devoted more or less time to talking with families, listened with more or less understanding, and diverged in judgment about the best way to handle patients.[4]

A few intensivists seemed to have eidetic (photographic) memories and could reel off relevant studies, percentages, and publications as they rounded. Some possessed formidable clinical acumen, an almost uncanny ability to determine when a patient's condition had altered. One man would enter a patient's room, sniff, and say, "he's bleeding," "she pooped," "his mouth stinks, I think he has something growing [a dangerous organism]." He was the only intensivist who invariably looked at the patient as well as the X rays and numbers, emphasizing to the residents the importance of what he half-mockingly called a "retinal scan." He would come into a room, question the assembled residents and fellows about the patient's condition, then say, "Look in his eyes." When no one moved, he'd repeat in a more commanding tone, "Look in his eyes!" Someone would open the patient's eyes and report that his pupils were pinpoints. "Exactly!" this man would say.[5]

The differences between attending physicians were so marked that one young fellow, early on in his fellowship, pulled me aside to ask, in a tone of distress, if I felt there was a great difference between the attendings. When I said yes, they seemed to do everything differently, from teaching to talking to patients to decision making, he seemed relieved to have his judgment validated.

The differences began with morning rounds. One man arrived precisely on the minute, at 7:30, and began immediately. Another was routinely 20 to 30 minutes late (this delay extended to most of his overstressed schedule, and hospital personnel learned to allow for it), while still another frequently telephoned after 30 to 45 minutes, saying he was unavoidably delayed and asking the fellows to begin without him.

Some attendings were conscientious about teaching during rounds, encouraging residents to express their opinions, citing statistics and studies; the pocket of one man's lab coat bulged with reprints from medical journals, which he distributed when a resident expressed interest. Another asked for opinions and citations, and employed the surgical technique of "teaching by humiliation." I noted one such occasion in my fieldnotes:

> [The intensivist] was questioning [a surgical resident] about some orders he had written [for medications], asking him how much of a dose his order would compute as, and what was the recommended dose, etc. "Don't you like the guy?" he asked, "Why are you trying to assassinate him?" When he

finished, the other two surgical residents laughed quietly to each other, it seemed to me, in relief that it was [this resident] rather than one of them.

Another intensivist raced through rounds with no teaching, telling residents what was wrong and what he wanted done for each patient. Two men received frequent calls on their cell phone; one seemed to be receiving medical calls that he disposed of rapidly; the other was obviously receiving nonmedical calls, for which he would interrupt rounds and leave the group to answer, conversing for some time on the phone. Since this man was easygoing when off the phone, allowing events to unfold rather than directing them so that the group moved rapidly from bed to bed, his rounds were extremely time consuming. (Many of his cell phone calls appeared to be associated with a wine bar he had opened, about which the nurses made frequent pointed jokes behind his back.)[6]

There was similar variation in the way attendings talked to patients, especially those conscious enough to be aware of the interaction. Some said nothing; others used a patronizing tone, as though talking to a young child or someone who was slightly feebleminded. Still others talked directly to patients, using the same tone of voice they used with everyone else. Not surprisingly, those who showed consideration in one area—arriving on time, making scrupulous efforts to teach residents, balancing the length of rounds against teaching, making the rounds as educational as possible without being oppressively long—were the men who were thoughtful and kind with patients. Their demeanor and behavior communicated caring and respect. I will quote my fieldnotes about one such intensivist:

> One patient reached for [his] hand, while he was examining her. He saw it, grasped the hand, and talked to her in a kind, compassionate tone, not in the least condescending, explaining that they plan to remove the breathing tube if she breathes well.
> The term "good" describes Baxter [the intensivist], in the biblical sense. He teaches with such care . . . he clearly feels responsible for [the residents'] learning during the SICU rotation. . . . When we rounded [on a patient with pneumonia] he asked her nurse, "Do you have anything to add?" He did this with several nurses. He respects himself and others.

On the other hand, the attending who called day after day to say that he was unavoidably detained, and then held exceptionally long rounds interrupted by frequent nonmedical telephone calls, was the doctor who spoke patronizingly to patients, and who left the room in the middle of an end-of-life meeting with a dying patient's family to respond to a call on his cell phone. The demeanor of the young intensivist who had been a resident and fellow in the medical center was particularly interesting: He had obviously observed his seniors and consciously adopted the most effective practices of each.[7]

The surgeon-head of the SICU contended that the variation in the practices of intensivists was a source of strength when treating gravely ill patients. He wrote: "The attending rotation schedule, criticized by Cassell, is in fact a useful tool that automatically generates independent second opinions concerning patients whose survival appears unlikely."[8] On this, he and I disagree. Dissimilarity in clinical philosophies may be helpful in generating "independent second opinions" when caring for patients who survive their stay in the unit; however, there is no way that dissimilarity in care and compassion when dealing with dying patients and their families can be effective.

Perhaps the greatest variation among attendings was how they treated terminal patients. At a nurses' meeting, one nurse spoke derisively of how patients' conditions might "change" when a new attending came on service. A patient can be "dying," one week, then another intensivist arrives and declares "I'm going to save that person," and they are no longer dying, she declared, noting that the following week, when a third attending came on service, the patient might well become "dying" again. (When I remarked that I generally ask a nurse about prognoses, that the patient's nurse generally seems to know whether or not someone is going to survive, she responded: "Yes, we know, but this is a gut feeling that can't be measured, so the doctors pay no attention.")[9]

The best nurses seemed to know not only the patients' prognoses, but also a great deal about the attending physicians.[10] Whenever I wanted to verify an observation or hunch, I would consult a few exceptionally intelligent and observant nurses who would verify or contradict my impression. Naturally, they must have known far more about me than I realized, and it took time before the nurses trusted me sufficiently to speak honestly and openly. This was one of the benefits of spending 18 months conducting research in the Midwest unit, an advantage I lacked in Texas and New Zealand.[11]

No Man Is a Hero . . .

An academic luminary needs a support system: competent laboratory assistants to conduct research when he is absent, fulfilling other responsibilities. A secretary to keep track of his schedule, making appointments and travel arrangements, holding off importunate callers—be they students, colleagues, administrators, or reporters. The more dazzling the star, the more capable the secretary must be to keep track of his multiple responsibilities and hectic schedule, tactfully reminding him where he is supposed to be and when—and devising credible excuses when he is late or does not show up. A devoted wife who sympathizes with his goals, understands the pressures buffeting him, and is willing to pick up the pieces when he is unable to fulfill his social and familial responsibilities (this ranges from sending cards and gifts to *his* relatives, holding dinner parties that he may not attend, and pacifying resentful children who complain that they never see their father). Residents and fellows with the ability to care for patients on their own and with enough self-confidence to know when to call for help. Skilled nurses who carry out the attending physician's treatment decisions and are intelligent enough to know when *not* to obey that doctor's instructions, going up the chain of command to a superior or, when necessary, notifying the attending, himself, that someone's condition has seriously deteriorated and that he would do well to observe that patient in person as soon as possible.

One particularly dazzling luminary observed plaintively: "My life is managed by women, so I can manage men!"

I am speaking as though the star were a man, with crucial members of the support system being women. This is most frequently the case.[12] The dynamics differ with a female star, and it is an unusual woman able to negotiate the relationships and complexities of medical stardom: commanding without alienating nurses, directing subordinates while conducting research, delegating responsibilities to competent aides, achieving a working bond with a secretary—steering between resentment from or victimization by her[13]—and fulfilling parental and spousal responsibilities.[14]

Although secretaries and wives may discuss the star's foibles, a certain code of loyalty may keep such talk within bounds. No such code restrains nurses, who share information and impressions with one another during working hours and when they socialize after work. Moreover, nurses have direct access to the hospital "grapevine," communicating frequently with colleagues and friends in other departments. The SICU attendings might have been surprised at how clearly they were perceived by the nurses and how much the nurses knew about each. Speculations about marital disharmony, possible affairs, lay psychiatric diagnoses ("he didn't take his lithium today"), and actual as opposed to self-convinced sexual orientation, were shared. The view from below, of dominant men by subordinate women, can be almost terrifyingly acute.

In this respect, the relationship of male stars to their female support system is not unique. The efforts, self-view and, on occasion, pretensions of the men contrast markedly with the way they are perceived by the women who may, nevertheless, publicly support both the men's efforts and their self-importance. An anthropological example, the Munduracú, an Amazonian Indian tribe, comes to mind. When first studied by the anthropologist Robert Murphy, he described the myths that recount how in the old days the men, confined to a subordinate role by the dominant women, achieved control by wresting away the *karoko*, or sacred flutes or trumpets, then keeping all knowledge of the instruments and the rituals based on them from the now-subordinated women. Murphy's early writings emphasized the subordinate status of Munduracú women and their ignorance of what went on in the men's house where the instruments were hidden and played. Twenty years later, when he and his wife, who conducted fieldwork with him, wrote a book about the Munduracú women, it emerged that the women knew a good bit about the instruments and were "obviously less impressed with male prowess and its props than were the men."[15] It also emerged that although the men's ideology, rituals, and practices emphasized the central role of men's hunting, which is central to their religion and spirit world, it appears that gardening, the bulk of which is done by women, provides a larger proportion of the tribe's food. Hunting is more highly valued, meat is more sought after by women as well as men, but the women's work in providing as well as preparing food is utterly essential. Moreover, it is the women, working together in groups, who gossip and "exchange valuable information about people."[16]

"That Was Not on My Watch"

With the exception of one intensivist, who had experience working with the other senior attendings as a resident and fellow, none of the intensivists knew exactly how his colleagues practiced, nor did anyone seem to want to know. Naturally, an attending physician who came on call on a Monday morning and found a backlog of patients whom he believed had no hope of survival would have notions of what his predecessor did and did not do. Talking to families could be equally enlightening; if family members indicated that no one had said a word to them the previous week, the absence of interaction was revealing. But publicly, the intensivists denied knowledge—and responsibility— for what had occurred when someone else was on call. There seemed no sense of corporate responsibility, not even among the two co-directors of the unit. "That was not on my watch!" was the phrase I heard more than one attending utter when complaints arose about the behavior of a colleague.

The fact that each intensivist was, in some sense, "in business for himself" is consonant with the individualistic, capitalist moral economy of the United States. This offered a striking contrast to the consensual moral economy observed among intensivists in socialist New Zealand. These differences will be explored in subsequent chapters.

I observed no evidence of a team spirit among the Midwest SICU intensivists. Underlying the efficient functioning of many institutions is team bonding, or what social scientists refer to as primary group loyalties. In American hospitals, such bonding is being attacked from many different directions. Insofar as physicians are encouraged toward part-time work and responsibility, and to visualize their futures apart from the institution, humane and sensitive patient care suffers.

Serving the Community and Saving Lives in Texas

The open SICU I studied in Texas was run by trauma surgeons. They cared for the trauma patients and helped coordinate care for the other patients, who were followed by the surgeon who had operated on them.

Money and an ethic of billable hours appeared relatively inconsequential to these men. Although there was talk of upgrading the hospital to make it more attractive to wealthier patients, everyone seemed aware of the hospital's mission to take care of their own community, which included a large number of relatively impoverished Hispanic families. This mission gave the trauma surgeons power and prestige in the hospital and in the region, where the county hospital had the only civilian Level 1 trauma service in south Texas.

The moral economy of the hospital and the trauma surgeons was centered on serving the community and saving lives. Each of the surgeons seemed to speak at least some Spanish, a necessity in a community where half the inhabitants were Hispanic, and all appeared devoted to waging the surgical battle against death. It was clear that the trauma surgeons loved the challenge and excitement of trauma, with constant emergencies and dramatic "saves."[17] At a weekly meeting on trauma deaths, an attending told me that many surgeons do not want to specialize in trauma: A surgeon can go into private practice and perform elective procedures, hernias, and gallbladders, and sleep nights (instead of being on call every fifth night), and make more money than a trauma surgeon. "But you'd be bored," I responded, and another attending indicated that this was why they were there.

I never quite figured out the ICU schedule of the three trauma surgeons who acted as intensivists; it appeared to be catch-as-catch-can, with morning rounds conducted by one in a somewhat unpredictable fashion. The timing of rounds was unpredictable as well, with residents and medical students cooling their heels, waiting for rounds to begin anytime between 8:00 A.M. to noon. This was difficult for the residents, who said that they could not start many procedures on patients until after the intensivist had determined what should be done for each patient during morning rounds. My fieldnotes observed:

> Everyone was hanging around and hanging around waiting for rounds to begin. They told me they come in about 7:00 and check the numbers for the Critical Care Patient Worksheet. They do some procedures, but nothing big, because rounds might interrupt it. . . . Rounds today did not begin until 10:59! Exhausting for the residents to have to come in early and then hang around.

One resident asked if they waited around like this at the Midwest medical center and I responded that they did not. Rounds there usually began with the X rays at about 7:30 A.M., 8:00 at the latest, and although one intensivist was habitually late, he would telephone and direct the fellows to begin without him. As a graduate student conducting research in the Blue Mountains of Jamaica, I learned that events began whenever all the participants had gathered and felt ready, often several hours later than scheduled; this was referred to laughingly as "Jamaican time." A similar phenomenon, labeled "Indian time," has been noted among American Indians.[18] Was "Texas time" observed in this SICU alone, in south Texas, or in a wider geographic area? Perhaps the fact that the trauma surgeon-intensivists had to respond to constant unscheduled emergencies at any time of day or night accounted for the irregularity of rounds.

Although I was told that the trauma surgeon-intensivists occasionally "butted heads" with other surgical specialists, I observed no conflict stemming from a bed shortage, which, in this hospital, resulted from a scarcity of nurses to staff the ICU beds they actually possessed. The spacious state-of-the-art unit contained three "pods," only two of which were in use.[19] An ICU nurse said that it was her job to decide every morning whether operative procedures should be canceled because of a lack of usable beds. (She reported how a vascular surgeon, upset about cancellation of his operation, inquired: "What if this were President Bush?" and she responded, "If it were President Bush, I'd work a double shift!") When unexpected trauma cases arrived, with too few staffed beds for them, the chief, who was head of trauma and the SICU, made the final decision.

Unlike the Midwest unit, where I observed no sense of corporate responsibility among the intensivists, the five trauma surgeons evinced a strong esprit de corps. The men ranged in age from early thirties to early forties, with a relatively young chief, who appeared thoughtful, considerate, and extremely knowledgeable—belying the macho, devil-may-care surgical stereotype. One man said that they try to set up ways to work together comfortably for the next 20 years: the surgeon who preferred the ER spent more time there, the man who favored trauma concentrated on that, and the other three rotated in a somewhat unpredictable fashion in the ICU. One of the three acted as ICU "fellow," working as a trauma surgeon after 4:00 P.M. (He reported that when an emergency erupted, he occasionally had to look at his watch to see whether he was a critical care fellow or trauma surgeon.)

Although the Texas surgeons seemed well versed in the critical care literature, citing relevant articles and statistics when teaching residents and medical students, no one conducted basic research. They did carry out clinical studies organized by a competent and efficient research nurse. Despite the fact that these men appeared familiar with, and apparently practiced "evidence-based medicine," it did not appear to be subscribed to with the same quasi-religious "act of devotion" as in the Midwest Center.[20] Their pride seemed less focused on academic proficiency than on practical efficacy, on saving lives, and serving their community.

5

Is Death the Enemy, or Suffering?

Diverging Moral Economies

The Midwest SICU is semi-closed. Responsibility for patient care is shared between the surgeon who operated on the patient (referred to as the primary attending) and the intensivist on call that particular week. Conflict erupted, on occasion, when an intensivist proposed to shift a patient from "cure" to "comfort care" against the adamant opposition of the patient's surgeon.

The surgeons, as a rule, hated to let a dying patient go. A surgeon might tell family members there was no reason to worry, when an intensivist had warned them that the patient's condition was grave. I repeatedly witnessed disagreement between the two parties about patients' prognoses and the correct course of action. With a patient who seemed irrevocably in terminal decline, the intensivists would propose discontinuing aggressive treatment; the surgeon would insist that the patient was going to survive, refusing to endorse a shift to comfort care. Gradually, I realized that the two specialties subscribed to radically different moral economies.[1] Unrecognized by the conflicting parties, these ethical differences led to miscommunication and delays that escalated costs when there were formidable odds against patient survival.

The Covenantal Ethic

Now therefore come thou, let us make a covenant (b'rith), I and thou. . . . The Lord watch between me and thee, when we are absent one from another.

—Genesis 31: 44–48

Surgeons define their relationship to the patient as a promise to battle death on that person's behalf. During a complex and difficult operation, a colleague remarked to the surgeon, "You know that logo with Sir Lancelot on a horse carrying a sword. Well, we should have you on a horse with a scalpel."[2] The enemy the surgeon-warrior confronts is the Grim Reaper.

The notion of *covenant* emerges from the biblical Scriptures where it defines the relationship between God and his people; it may then also characterize the relationship of two parties. "At the heart of a covenant is an exchange of promises, an agreement that shapes the future between two parties," explains theologian William F. May.[3] Although the concepts of covenant and contract are related, in spirit they are quite different:

> Contracts involve buying and selling; covenants involve giving and receiving. Contracts are external; covenants are internal to the parties involved. Contracts are signed to be expediently discharged; covenants have a gratuitous, growing edge to them that nourishes rather than limits relationship. Contracts can be filed away, but a covenant becomes part of one's history and shapes in unexpected ways one's self perception and perhaps even destiny.[4]

The surgeon–patient covenant, then, involves an implicit promise to the patient: I will not abandon you; I will battle death for you; our relationship involves giving and receiving; it is a deeper and stronger commitment than money can buy; such commitment is part of my identity as a surgeon.

I described the notion of the surgeon–patient covenant to a woman surgeon with whom intensivists had had a number of explosive confrontations. She grasped the concept immediately, and spoke of her first meeting with a patient whom the ICU physicians had—against her adamant opposition—wanted to shift to comfort care: "I looked him in the eye and said, 'I'll take care of you,' and that was it."

"When someone comes into your office, you enter into a contract to cure them from their disease, to save them from what is trying to kill them," explained a physician who was both trauma surgeon and intensivist, "There's all this talk, which is justified, about the special relationship between surgeons and their patients, because you go inside their bodies and rearrange things permanently. And there can never be an error, there can never be a lapse in judgment. It has to be perfect every time."[5]

He noted that surgeons talk about foiling the Grim Reaper. The important thing was defeating death and getting the patient out of the hospital, even if to a nursing home. At this hospital they say, "No one wants to be a star on Tuesday afternoon—no one wants to have their case discussed and be the surgeon raked over the coals at the M & M." (At the weekly Mortality and Morbidity [M & M] conference, surgeons castigate colleagues who they feel did not do everything possible to save a patient.)[6] For surgeons the choice is simple: life or death. Examining the quality of that saved life is beside the point. If patients have a chance at living, it is wrong, even immoral, to deprive them of that chance.[7]

When a patient's death is discussed at the M & M conference, the surgeon is asked if he or she did everything possible to save that patient. The surgeon is *not* asked about the patient's subsequent fate. "One would rather have a live patient in a nursing home, potentially suffering—they're out of the hospital," said the trauma surgeon-intensivist. If the patient dies, the surgeon is "pulled over the coals" by colleagues, unless he or she shows that everything possible was done to save that person. No shame, however, attaches to "doing everything possible."[8]

Not doing everything possible, even at the patient's expressed wish, may disturb surgeons. A SICU fellow, trained as a surgeon, was upset when a patient indicated that he did not want an operation to insert a feeding tube and wanted the tube attached to his ventilator removed. The patient's wishes were followed, he was shifted to comfort care only, and his family made arrangements for him to be sent to a hospice near their home. The fellow could not accept the idea that someone could decide to forgo feeding when a simple feeding tube would keep him alive. (The condition of the severely handicapped patient had been deteriorating for some time, and it was obvious that this decline was intensifying.) The SICU fellow was unimpressed by the concept of autonomy, and by the fact that this 67-year-old man, who lived in a nursing home, had stopped enjoying life and had planned his own funeral in detail. Finally, I told him that as a surgeon, his job was to save people, and that this was good; he should feel that people should be saved; but that perhaps decisions about the end of life should not be made by surgeons who felt that their job was to save patients. He was able to accept this formulation.

Doing everything possible can, on occasion, be broadly defined. Of one dying patient in his eighties, whose metastatic cancer had led to the removal of his stomach, spleen, and other organs, my fieldnotes observed:

> Schnurr [the surgeon] is still saying we're in cure mode, not comfort. "We're still flogging him," said Courtney [a surgical resident].[9] "That's just the term I use in my notes," I told her. Sumner [the intensivist] said: "My guess is that we're a few days away from withdrawing care, no matter what the family says.[10] The patient is going downhill and the decision will be made for them." "God will decide the problem," said Sumner. Courtney thinks Schnurr is being so difficult because he's mad at himself for operating in the first place. Turns out he came in Saturday and made a screaming scene in front of the residents.

Screaming scenes are not unknown among surgeons, many of whom have the reputation of being prima donnas and who are often described by OR nurses as being "high strung"—at least the men are so described, the women are labeled "bitches." An intensive care physician who e-mailed me a description of one such scene, where a fellow was screamed at and blamed for a patient's postoperative bleeding, noted:

> This behavior once again typifies the misdirected and disproportionate rage that characterizes many surgeons' responses to unexpected, adverse events.

When I asked the fellow at whom this scene was directed what happened, he said of Dr. Friedlich, the surgeon: "He was beyond yelling. He went ballistic!" The surgeon screamed at the fellow, demanding that he, himself, leave the unit to fetch blood from the blood bank, which the fellow refused to do, saying he had responsibility for all the ICU patients. The fellow told me that he heard that Dr. Friedlich had recently had several instances of postoperative bleeding in a row.

"Surgeons are bad at dealing with their own complications," said a transplant surgeon. "If I were in charge, I'd have others fix it. You have a sense of personal ownership and want to ignore complications." A New Zealand cardiac-care intensivist made a similar point, remarking that when a surgeon refused to recognize that one of his patients was going to die, he had to then appeal to the chief in order to shift the patient from heroic to comfort care: "Surgeons are magical about their own patients, but highly rational about the patients of other surgeons," he noted.

The surgeon who "went ballistic" with the fellow had a history of angry confrontations with the SICU fellows and attendings. Of one of his patients, my fieldnotes observe:

> Yesterday, Dr. Friedlich said of Mr. Green (who has been lying there with his mouth wide open for weeks now, looking just about dead) that he may be septic, but we can treat that; he's better now than a week ago; and that the patient wants to continue care if there's any hope, and there is hope. He's been here 2½ weeks. If he does get better, he'd have to go to rehab, then have another operation, recover from that, go to rehab, etc. And he's 73. . . . His living will, which is just about useless, said [the ICU attending] says, don't continue if it's hopeless. But how does one define hope? Friedlich clearly defines it differently than most of the ICU docs. [The patient's] daughter had told [the nurse] that his wife had died recently after a long drawn-out illness and he said he didn't want that. But Friedlich says this guy doesn't have a fatal disease. He has fungal sepsis, but he can get over that.

Two days later, the intensivist on call that week told me that he had talked with the daughter for an hour by telephone. She told him that this conversation was the first time anyone had informed her what survival for her father would entail; she knew he would need another operation, but she did not know he would have to spend a long time in rehab, learning to walk again, and other rehabilitative activities, as well, before having the second operation, which would probably follow the same course. The evening after he talked with the daughter, said the intensivist, the patient had a neurological consult, and although the neurologist had said nothing to him, he discovered that he had told the surgeon that the patient was quadriplegic—possibly from a stroke. Some of the residents knew about the quadriplegia, others did not, but no one had informed the SICU attending. In any case, said the intensivist, the daughter had the *cujones* to obtain his pager number, which he never gives patients; she paged him and asked, "I want to withdraw care, do I have to come in?" "Yes," said the attending, who had never met her. She made her father DNR (do not resuscitate) and he died two days later.

The trauma surgeon who was also an intensivist described an occurrence when a patient on whom he had operated was deteriorating in the SICU while he kept pushing for more time, rather than withdrawing therapy and shifting to comfort care. Finally, the surgeon-head of the unit put him on the spot, inquiring, "Let's say you were the ICU attending for this patient, how would you handle this?" He then realized that he had done none of the things with the patient and his family that he did as an intensivist, because that had seemed contrary to his goal as surgeon, which was "to cure them [patients] regardless of the cost." For a surgeon, "failure is not acceptable," he said. "As long as you have a beating heart in a nursing home somewhere, you are successful."[11]

The head of the ICU, who had pointed out the contradiction between the behaviors of the man as trauma surgeon and as intensivist, went the extra mile himself for a man on whom he had operated. The patient had shot another man at close range, standing over his victim, pumping bullets into him, until he himself was blasted by a police officer. The police discovered that the patient/killer lived in a distant city and had apparently been recruited to carry out the killing. The killer ended up in the ICU, where the surgeon-head suggested employing an experimental technology to increase his chance of survival. "We could get 'compassionate use,'" argued the surgeon-head. "'Compassionate use!' exploded a colleague, "for a murderer?"

Unlike behavior, which can be observed directly, motives are murky. One might speculate that the temperament of those who go into surgery, supported by the methods used to train surgical recruits,[12] involves a sense of unworthiness or "inner shame" that is defended against by a drive to be the best, a need to be perfect. A patient's death, then, must be fought to the bitter end, since it reveals to the world the unworthiness of the surgeon.[13] "Failure" as the trauma surgeon-intensivist observed, "is not acceptable." One might also speculate that surgery increases the patient's risk of death as well as increasing pain and suffering at least for a day or two. It is perhaps easier for a surgeon not to operate and accept that the patient has a fatal condition than to operate, find the same thing, and then have to "let go" without having "fully atoned" for the increase in pain and suffering wrought by the knife and the scissors, the clamps and the retractors. Consequently, it is much harder to "let go" when one has "breached the boundaries of the skin" than when one has not.[14]

Who "Owns" the Patient?

Surgeons do not speak of a covenant with the patient (that is my interpretation) but rather of a sense of ownership. The transplant surgeon who stated that he would prefer to have others fix his complications, nonetheless took exception to the proprietary attitudes of the intensivists. Discussing the resultant conflicts, he said:

> I feel the ownership. . . . Who owns the patient there [in the ICU] is a big issue. In many cases they (ICU attendings) feel that *they* own the patient. I think that's really wrong. These people (patients) didn't come, didn't get referred to the ICU at ____ Hospital (he laughs), they got referred to a vascular surgeon or a transplant surgeon.[15]

Ownership refers to a sense of personal responsibility, routinely going the extra mile to make sure that the patient is properly cared for. Surgery is the ultimate hands-on specialty: the surgeon's hands pierce the envelope of skin, entering and violating the secret recesses of the body, attempting to repair the ravages of disease or malfunction. "The soul's in there, somewhere" remarked one surgeon, discussing the intimacy of the surgical relationship. The use of the term "ownership" by the transplant surgeon goes beyond that intimacy toward an entailed consequence: the power of the professional to make final decisions about what should be done to and for that patient.[16]

Suggesting that others should fix the complications while insisting on retaining the final decision-making ability would sound a dissonance between responsibility and authority. The dissonance may come from the fact that the first statement is relatively abstract: Others should fix any complications, which presumptively are minor; but should these be severe, then they can be judged as a statement of failure, which the surgeon has difficulty in accepting. On the other hand, the second statement is concrete and specific: No one is going to tell me what should be done to *my* patients, with whom I have a covenantal relationship and to whom I have a special responsibility. Whether one calls these attitudes "magical" or "covenantal," the fact remains that most surgeons find it almost unbearable to acknowledge defeat in their battle with the Grim Reaper and have great difficulty abandoning heroic measures at what might be—in the judgment of other doctors—the end of a patient's life.

A disproportionate number of the conflicts I witnessed in the SICU were between transplant surgeons and intensivists. This is not a random occurrence. Transplant surgeons often know a patient for years before that person obtains a transplant, and they care for that patient from then onward. "We're their primary care physicians," explained one. Naturally, their feeling of ownership is far more powerful than that of say, a trauma surgeon, who may not meet a patient until that person is carried into the ER gravely injured. The strength of the relationship, influenced by time and mutual interaction, determines the power of the covenant. (Interestingly, I was told by a nurse that similar disagreements may occur when patients are dying in the neighboring medical ICU, between the private doctor, who may have known that person for some time, and the medical intensivist.)[17]

When I witnessed conflict between surgeons and intensivists, they often seem to be talking past one another. It is not that one is correct and the other wrong; one ethical, the other unprincipled. They subscribe to two utterly different ethics or moral economies.

Allocating Scarce Resources and Averting Suffering

It was Friday. The Midwest SICU was full. There were no empty beds for the trauma cases that were likely to come in during the weekend. An intensivist, discussing a surgeon who flatly refused to have a patient in her eighties moved from the SICU, finding every excuse possible—including some that sounded preposterous[18]—said: "Well our viewpoints differ. I see an ICU with room for the 18 sickest patients. He just sees his patient for whom he wants the very best."

Although the view of the intensivist could be classified as "utilitarian" ethics, as did Zussman in his 1992 study of medical ethics and intensive care, I prefer a more specific classification, reflecting the problem of how to distribute a limited resource among members of a community—indeed, a moral economy—rather than thinking in the abstract principles of "the greatest happiness to the greatest number."[19]

The issue of how a scarce resource should be allocated comes closer to the reasoning of intensivists. Zussman, whose field research in ICUs began in 1985, observes that the questions posed by scarcity of medical resources are still novel to American medicine.[20] They are surely less novel today, although as compared to other countries, we still adhere to practices and values based on abundance.[21]

Zussman plotted the relation between the number of empty beds in the two American ICUs he studied and the length of stay for each patient; in each, patients were discharged after shorter stays when empty beds were scarce.[22] A transplant surgeon mentioned a related phenomenon. He asserted that when beds were in short supply, the intensive care physicians pressed him to discuss end–of–life issues with patients' families. He said:

> Just because all the beds in the ICU are filled, to me is not necessarily the
> burning platform that leads me to have a conversation that afternoon with

someone. I may not be ready, or the other people I work with may not be ready, the nurses may not be ready, the family may not be ready. . . . This might not be taking the global view of it, but on the micro level, just because there is an ICU bed shortage doesn't mean that that's the right time or moment to have that conversation with the family about what we're going to do.[23]

Zussman noted that the (what he termed "utilitarian") principle of triage was not applied in an evenhanded fashion in the medical ICUs he studied. My observations support his, although the factors he listed that biased its practice did not parallel the ones I observed. Zussman's factors were: (1) a predisposition in favor of excluding patients who were "not sick enough" while retaining patients who were "too sick" to benefit from the services of the unit, (2) an attachment to some, but not all, families, and (3) the continued presence in intensive care of private physicians.[24]

Zussman's second and third factor had little apparent influence in the two American units I observed. Although nurses and on occasion residents in the units I studied clearly preferred some well-spoken and obviously devoted families to others, whom they characterized as difficult and abusive, I did not observe intensive care attendings making important decisions based on this preference.[25] One might consider the occasionally conflictual relation between surgeons and intensivists in the semi-closed surgical unit as roughly analogous to Zussman's third factor; this, however, omits *decision-making power*. The shared authority of surgeons and intensivists in the surgical unit complicated decision making in a more overt fashion than did the relations between private and intensive care physicians in the hospitals Zussman studied, where, so far as I could tell, the official (if not always actual) decision-making power was assigned to the intensivists.[26]

More than scarce resources are involved in the intensivists' relation to patients. When I questioned the trauma-surgeon-intensivist, who said his goal as a surgeon was curing the patient regardless of the cost, about his goal as an intensivist, he responded: "I think the goal for the intensivist is not cure, and not beating off the Grim Reaper regardless of cost, but embracing the implicit contract with the patient to do the best thing for the patient." He added, "that goal is different than to have the patient live and get out of the hospital, whatever it takes." He continued:

You make a deal, I'm not going to say with the Devil, because I would never say that, you make a deal with the Reaper . . . in the sense that you know death is going to occur . . . and tell the Grim Reaper, so to speak, "You can have this one, but it's on my terms."

He drew an interesting comparison, saying the surgeon's approach was "paternalistic": "I will protect you, I will beat off all the enemies" as opposed to a more "maternalistic" intensivists' approach. "A mother would never want her child to suffer," he declared.[27] In this moral economy, needless suffering rather than death per se is the enemy.

Crucial Decisions

The weekly shift in intensive care physicians in the Midwest SICU, each with a different practice style, choice of drugs, and patterns of decision making, was exacerbated by a certain ambiguity about who had the power to make fateful decisions, such as whether and when to shift a patient from heroic to comfort care. The shared responsibility between surgeons and intensivists, with diverging moral economies, led to perplexities (when patients' families might be given contradictory messages by surgeons and intensivists), disagreement, and, on occasion, conflict.

Let me note that the operating surgeon, with fixed ideas about what should and should not be done for his or her patient, did not change; the same surgeon remained the primary attending while the intensivist on service rotated weekly. We might hazard a guess that surgeons would be encouraged to adamantly insist on a particular course of action, hoping that the following week they might be dealing with a more "cooperative" intensivist. We might also speculate that intensivists might be tempted to pass along (or "punt") problematic patients, whose situation involved conflict of one sort or another, to next week's on-call colleague. Such handing over responsibility might not even be entirely conscious. In the event of a difficult decision, such as whether a patient's prognosis should be judged hopeless, it would be all too easy to rationalize postponement, resolving that the situation required additional time and information.

Naturally, one may argue—as did one SICU attending physician—that conflict between surgeon and attending, although painful, had its benefits. He felt that having the surgeon act as "the patient's advocate," holding out for life at any cost, forced the intensivist to reflect carefully before broaching the subject of a shift from cure to comfort care.

When disagreement between surgeons and intensivists erupted

about whether and when it was time to shift a patient to comfort care, it was unclear who had the responsibility for the final decision. In the situations I observed, it seemed to me that the person, whether surgeon or intensivist, who possessed the greatest personal and political crunch was the one whose opinion prevailed. Thus, force of character, reputation, and rank in the medical center affected these decisions

What also influenced end-of-life decisions was the willingness and ability to fight low-down and dirty when necessary. One highly moral, caring intensivist did not seem to have the stomach for this kind of street-fighting, nor did he seem able to speak directly to families about the necessity to let the patient go. Although he knew when a patient was terminal, and would speak of it being time to move to comfort care, this man would often use technical terms when talking to families that would be easy for them to misunderstand,[28] or show them a patient's suppurating wound so that they, themselves, might make the decision to discontinue aggressive therapy. This kind, gentle man also seemed unwilling or unable to go to the mat with the operating surgeon. "Dr. Baxter does not like to deal with death," said a nurse, "I don't think he knows this; he *thinks* he deals with it." A few other intensivists would discuss the issue with family members and then, if necessary, do battle with surgeons who refused to acknowledge that a patient had little if any hope of surviving. When intensivists and families did decide to focus on comfort alone, removing ventilator support to allow a terminal patient to die, surgeons frequently made remarks such as "I am not Dr. Kevorkian!" and "I will not help you kill this patient!"

Intensivists differed on what one doctor called their "level of comfort" in deciding that it was time to abandon hope of survival. One man seemed relatively unconflicted; he raised the subject earlier than his colleagues, asking family members what the patient would have wanted and suggesting that prolonging death was neither kind nor practical. The surgeons detested this man's forthright approach and the speed with which he decided a patient's case was hopeless. I was told that some referred to him as "Doctor Death." Others, however, took far more time in defining a case as "hopeless," and had more apparent difficulty discussing these issues with family members or with the surgeons who had operated on that patient. The differences in level of comfort extended to the age of patients: I was told that one intensivist customarily abandoned hope for gravely ill patients over the age of 80. (These differences pose a striking contrast to the ICU

I studied in New Zealand, where all the intensivists discussed the matter and came to a consensual decision before proposing to shift a patient from heroic to comfort care.)

Recording end-of-life discussions between intensivists and family members, our research team found an enormous disparity not only in interactional styles, but also in the number of tapes obtained for each intensivist.[29] We managed to obtain only one recording of an interview held by one of the intensivists; it was our impression that this extremely private man did hold such meetings but abhorred being recorded. Another intensivist took part in two recorded interviews; other senior doctors were present at each, however, and this man did not direct the discussion. This is the doctor who, I was told, left an end-of-life discussion to answer a call on his cell phone. I attended a family meeting run by this intensivist that was not recorded.[30] On this occasion, he was cornered and almost forced to carry out a formal end-of-life interview, which he postponed for several hours, keeping family members in an extremely difficult, conflictual situation, waiting.[31] During the interview, he displayed ignorance of the problematic family situation, addressing his questions and remarks to a family member with apparent psychiatric difficulties, while ignoring the person with formal Power of Attorney, who had the legal ability to decide what should be done. We were unable to determine whether this man avoided end-of-life meetings with families, postponing decisions until the next intensivist came on service, or whether such discussions were carried out informally at times when no researcher was present to listen or record the meeting. In contrast, one conscientious attending, for whom we had a number of recordings, "joked" about the dying patients he inherited at the beginning of his week on-service; our team noticed that many of his end-of-life meetings with family members were conducted on Mondays or Tuesdays (the new attending began work early Monday morning), and we wondered whether he was conducting some of the interviews postponed by his colleagues.[32]

In our project's tape-recorded interviews, the Midwest intensivists made valiant attempts to speak English rather than medical-eese; nevertheless, much of their phraseology was medical and/or Latinate.[33] Also, compared with the family meetings I attended in New Zealand, the American doctors talked more. There seemed to be almost a fear of silence among the intensivists, who filled each pause with a torrent of words. The meetings were shorter, as well; the on-service doctors who held these interviews had other pressing responsibilities in the unit, and their tone of voice and body language often indicated the termination of an interview. I doubt that they were aware of this; doctors have perfected a way of wordlessly indicating that this talk is over that is so smooth that they, themselves, no longer realize they are utilizing these powerful communicative mechanisms.

I did not observe conflict at the end of life in the open Texas unit, where surgeons had final decision-making responsibility for the patients they operated on, nor in the closed New Zealand ICU, where medical responsibility for the patient was relinquished to the ICU attendings when the patient was accepted in the unit.[34] In Texas, the covenantal ethic prevailed. In New Zealand, on the other hand, the intensivists considered potential suffering (or "quality of life") and scarce resources when making crucial decisions.

The following chapter will show how these two moral economies play out at the end of life in the Midwest and Texas SICUs.

6

Confronting Death in the Surgical Intensive Care Unit

Fateful Decisions in the Midwest SICU

Almost all the patients in the Midwest SICU were highly sedated.[1] Their awareness levels were measured by a "Ramsay Score," rating a patient's condition from "cooperative, oriented and tranquil," through "anxious, or agitated and restless," to "no response" or "unable to assess."[2]

The co-director of the SICU said that they administer narcotics and sedatives[3] to relieve anxiety and put the patient to sleep. He argues that it is so excruciating to be awake in the SICU, attached to tubes and with a breathing tube down one's throat, that it is kinder for the intensivists to sedate patients. Some of the drugs they administer have an amnesiac effect as well, so that patients subsequently remember nothing of what happened; often, they do not even remember the unit. When former patients take what the staff call their "victory lap" (where a patient returns to the unit to thank the doctors and nurses who saved his or her life, slowly walking from one end to the other to the plaudits of everyone there), many say that they remember nothing about their time in the SICU. Another SICU physician reported that there is a great deal of literature indicating that patients who remember the ICU experience—of not being able to talk, having tubes emerging from every orifice, and being unable to communicate that they are in pain because they have a tube down their throats—have, at best, bad memories of the ICU and, at worst, a kind of posttraumatic stress disorder. A third intensivist explained that the SICU patients are frequently septic after abdominal surgery; liver or kidney failure leads to a feverish, delirious patient who thrashes about; since the SICU nurses must care for two patients, a patient may struggle and dislodge tubes and get into trouble when the nurse is in the other room.[4]

In the New Zealand unit I studied, patients were generally awake. An Auckland intensivist was skeptical when told that the co-director of the Midwest SICU believes that the sedation keeps patients from remembering their time in the unit; he is too much of a scientist to accept that, he said. Their patients with whom they do follow-up interviews, do not remember their time in the unit either, and before accepting the contention of the Midwest intensivist, he would like to see a controlled study, comparing highly sedated and nonsedated patients showing that higher sedation alters memory or anything else. Another New Zealand intensivist reported that the Auckland patients are sedated at specific times for specific reasons, for example, when a percutaneous tracheotomy is performed at the bedside. During morning rounds, after a construction worker complained of pain—a three-ton block had dropped upon him—I told an intensivist that in the Midwest unit, he might be given Propofol. "Oh, amnesia juice!" he responded, explaining that they do not administer such drugs because then the patient is flat on his back and motionless and, as a result, far more likely to get pneumonia.[5] When I indicated that they give Propofol frequently in the Midwest unit, he commented, "Well, maybe they don't like to see patients awake." Instead, this patient was given an epidural, which anesthetized the painful area, rather than a sedative to put him to sleep.[6] Unlike the somnolent SICU patients, the construction worker was wide awake, joking with the doctors at his bedside and flirting with the female intensivist.

While lacking the medical knowledge to evaluate these divergent courses of action, I note an unintended consequence of the Midwest SCIU policy. It is far easier to relate to a highly sedated patient—who is unable to interact freely with doctors and nurses and who responds only to commands or physical stimuli—as a *body* in need of repair, rather than as a *person*. In a unit run by surgeons and anesthesiologists, specialties not renowned for conversing with patients, a patient's inability to interact may be an advantage, even if not consciously perceived as such. The sense of "owning the patient" then, when it is felt, consists of owning the patient's body, since the personality of a sedated patient is not in evidence.

At the end of life, then, the Midwest SICU intensivists had little knowledge of what kind of person that patient was (except as reported by family members).

Delegated "Autonomy"

Autonomy is currently seen as so integral to medical decision-making that it is advocated as a guiding principle even in individuals who are no longer autonomous.[7]

When end-of-life decisions had to be made, the patient's family was consulted. During end-of-life meetings, most—although not all—SICU intensivists inquired what the patient would have wished. Many families, however, did not seem to know, and even when they knew, often seemed to ignore the patient's statements. Although a few families had discussed these issues, and made it clear what they wanted, and some had even filled out Living Wills and given Power of Attorney to someone else, most family members were woefully unprepared to make the agonizing decision to move a person they loved from heroic to comfort care. "He's going downhill but you can't pull the plug on your brother," said one man, in a situation where his brother had made it clear before entering the hospital what course of action he favored, going so far as to plan his own funeral service.

When they consulted families, the intensivists spoke of "autonomy." I have doubts, however, about such "surrogate autonomy." For family members, suffused with grief and terror in the alien moonscape of the SICU, it seemed cruel to ask them to decide to "pull the plug on your brother." Was this really autonomy—or was it a kind of Pontius Pilate washing of hands, absolving the intensivist of a fateful and agonizingly difficult decision? (Also, let me note, absolving the intensivist and the hospital of potential lawsuits by any family member who might prefer to have the body "flogged" to the bitter end.)[8]

Let me present a few cases to give some idea of the variation in family constellations and responses of members.

"As Natural a Part of Living as Anything"

I will quote liberally from my fieldnotes, although some details have been changed in the interests of privacy. This note comes from a patient's early days in the unit.

> Mrs. Dalziel has pancreatic cancer. Everyone seems to think her prognosis is very poor, but her husband doesn't understand this, and the primary docs [the surgeons] only answer questions he asks and said Gina [a nurse] he doesn't know enough to ask the right questions.

The following day, the patient seemed alert, and the issue was whether to give her a tracheotomy.[9] The surgeon presented the odds to the family; they could give her a tracheotomy, and with chemotherapy there is an 80 percent rate of "partial response."[10] During rounds, the intensivist on service, the only one I heard actively teach the SICU residents what could and should be done in such situations, discussed what to do with a patient like Mrs. Dalziel who has a terminal diagnosis, yet is intubated [attached to a ventilator that breathes for her by a tube that goes down the throat]. He told them that the family agreed ahead of time that there should be no heroic measures, yet he noted that many family members find it hard to put the patient's desires ahead of their own. Family members often want to do everything possible because they can not bear to lose their loved one, even when the patient might prefer to stop treatment. Mrs. Dalzell will have a 40 percent chance of response in six weeks, but she cannot breathe now. How does one balance cure against comfort? There is the personal decision: Do you want to continue therapy? Then there is the medical decision, which is separate: Is further therapy futile?

The husband decided that patient should be given a tracheotomy to help her breathe, and almost two weeks later, my fieldnotes observed:

> Mrs. Dalziel has pneumonia, with green pus that can't be suctioned out. She has metastatic pancreatic cancer . . . the best response is 2 or 3 years "if she were perfect" said [the intensivist on service that week] . . . "if she didn't have all these other things wrong with her." Her sepsis has gotten dramatically worse in the past 24 to 48 hours.[11] [The intensivist presently on service] talked to Mr. Dalziel for an hour last night before she got so much worse. The best case scenario now would have her on the vent for months,[12] the worst, forever. Mr. Dalziel is coming in at noon. He said they talked it over and she doesn't want to be kept on machines. She's at home with the idea of dying; it's hard for him (I learned that they have five children from 6 to 14) but he doesn't want her coded.

Later the same day, my fieldnotes commented:

> We passed the Dalziels' room. Mr. Dalziel was sitting, holding his wife's hand. He did this all afternoon. His posture said to me that he was saying goodby to her.

A meeting with the husband was scheduled for late that afternoon. The intensivist, the surgeon who had operated on Mrs. Dalziel, and the nurse caring for the patient were in a little glass-fronted room used for such conferences. The recording system planned for these interviews was not yet in place, so we were unable to ask the husband's permission to record the meeting, and I felt it was disrespectful to take notes during the interview. (Afterward, I did record what occurred, however.) The surgeon spoke first:

> He wasn't as straightforward as [the intensivist], he found it difficult to say there was no hope. What he said . . . was that the chances for her recovery were going down. (I gather they were actually zero.) Mr. Dalziel was magnificent. Carla [the nurse] had told me that she'd never seen a family so well-prepared for death. He said "this is as natural a part of living as anything." He said they had been together 35 years and shared everything including five children, and that he was ready to go to just comfort measures. They discussed what to do: stop the blood pressure medicine, turn the ventilator down so that it was do longer doing the work of breathing for her. The husband just wanted to sit by her and hold her hand. He didn't want the children there, or a chaplain. . . . He just wanted to know if any of her organs could be donated, or if the cancer made this impossible. The doctors said she probably couldn't donate organs but [the intensivist] said they had a study on sepsis going, and perhaps she might be able to have some tissue taken for that. . . . "That would be wonderful!" said the husband, "She'd be thrilled." The intensivist said, "I don't know you as well as [the surgeon] but I think your wife was a very lucky woman to have you." "Oh, she was a blessing!" said the husband.

The Dalziels were obviously blessed in one another, but rarely is death in the SICU met with such courage and tranquility. More common are cases like the following.

"An Incredibly Heroic Operation"

We have already met Mr. Jan Bascombe, the 84-year-old African American patient who had his stomach, colon, spleen, and part of his pancreas removed because of metastatic cancer—and whose surgeon, Dr. Schnurr, threw a screaming fit in the unit. (A surgical resident had suggested that the surgeon was angry at himself for operating at all, and that was why he insisted on "flogging" a patient for whom there was obviously no hope.)

A nurse said that Mr. Bascombe was a drinker, alienated from his family for many years. The family situation was extremely complicated: an estranged wife—no one knew if they were still married; a daughter, who seemed to be in charge but who had not seen him for twenty years; a girlfriend, who did not know his current marital situation; other children; and many relatives who came to the unit inquiring: "Are they going to pull the plug on him?"

After 10 days in the ICU, the on-service intensivist scheduled a meeting with the patient's wife and family, explaining that the surgeon had not been able to remove all the cancer and that, at best, the patient had a few months to live. Mr. Bascombe, who had been taken off all sedatives, was not waking up, and the question was whether he had an abscess that, if drained, might give him a little more time, although the prognosis was hopeless. The wife, who had the authority to make a decision about discontinuing care, refused to decide, turning the issue over to their four children. Our team recorded a meeting with the family, where they said little—the intensivist did most of the talking—but asserted that they did not know what their father would have wanted.

On morning rounds, the intensivist pointed out that this man had chosen to have "an incredibly heroic operation," rather than going to a hospice; this may mean, he said, that he wants heroic treatment. He asked the group, consisting of residents, a fellow, and myself, whether we should try to get him off the "vent" [the ventilator that breathed for him] to give him a month or two at home. The fellow, a surgeon, said he thought that the operation was justified. The patient was bleeding to death, which is not a pleasant way to die, but that nothing more should be done to keep this gravely ill man alive, and doing more was both unethical and unjustified. The intensivist asked the residents and me what we thought: Should we stop his medications now or go on aggressively? I inquired about his family situation; talking as though he could go home for a month or two assumed that he had a loving family ready and willing to take him in, give him the messy and onerous care this dying cancer patient would require, and then sit by his bedside for a storybook death. The entire group was agreed: Stop now.

In the meantime, the surgeon had scheduled a full-body CT scan. Unless the scan showed metastases to the brain, he wanted to press ahead. The scan did not show metastases (although they may have been present, they were not visible on the scan), and the surgeon insisted they were still in "cure not comfort mode."

Twenty-two days after he arrived in the unit, Mr. Bascombe was still there. The story emerged at a SICU conference. The surgeon had finally agreed to do whatever the family decided, and the intensivist had met with the family. The daughter was the spokesperson; five family members were present, and they agreed to move the patient to comfort care. Two days later, reported the intensivist, another family meeting was held; all the first people had been forced out, and there was the daughter with thirty other relatives who had never come to the unit to visit. One man was in the daughter's face, literally—he was some sort of cousin or cousin's husband—who accused her of being a murderer and kept insisting, "Jesus doesn't want you to kill him!" The daughter finally gave in and said, "keep him alive." Later, she said to the intensivist, speaking of this group: "They're all crazy!"

After this stressful meeting, the daughter was unwilling to make a final decision, although earlier she had told a nurse and the social worker that her father would not want to be "hooked up to machines for the rest of his life." After discussing alternatives with the social worker, she decided to send the patient to an extended-care facility where, 10 days later, he was detached from the ventilator and died.

What was the cost of this "autonomy"—if indeed it could be defined as such? Leaving out the emotional costs, which had to be considerable, in terms of pain, sorrow, and guilt on the part of a family who had not seen the patient for many years, what was the cost in dollars and cents?[13] Of a complex and "incredibly heroic" operation that (according to an intensivist I consulted) "was unlikely to net him extra time in terms of being cancer free"?[14] Of at least 22 days in intensive care for a patient who everyone knew was terminal? Who paid?[15]

In an estranged family, one distant member insisting on life at any cost, using guilt and religion to blackmail the others, was able to increase the suffering and delay the inevitable death of an aged man who, all the doctors including his surgeon agreed, had a hopeless prognosis.

"Holding Out for a Miracle"

Some family members seem not only to hope for but to persist in waiting for miracles. Mrs. Corie Johnston is a good example. When the patient arrived in the unit, my fieldnotes observed:

> Mrs. Johnston is a 50 year old with a rectal abscess and necrotizing fasciitis, in acute renal failure. [The intensivist] said that two of the characteristics that predispose to this are obesity and diabetes.

This diabetic patient was, in fact, so obese that a nurse wondered if she had been able to walk before her hospitalization. Two days later, my notes observed that Mrs. Johnston's perirectal abscess had been debrided [the pus drained and dead skin cleaned out], and that the wound was enormous; her abscess extended from her buttocks up to her shoulder blades, penetrating down to the bone. The attending said that there was little hope of her surviving, and later, I learned that the surgeon who had cleaned up the wound had said: "She's dead."

Before being hospitalized, Mrs. Johnston had lived with her four children, in their late teens and early twenties, subsisting on a small disability pension. The following extract comes from my fieldnotes:

> She had I & D [incision and drainage] in the OR and at the bedside; the question is whether to try a colostomy and other radical procedures, or to give up, since her chance of survival is very small, possibly non-existent. The nurse said that when they clean her wound, they need to have lined baskets, because the transporters, who hold her open, vomit. "We have to go forward or withdraw," said [the intensivist]. Her family doesn't realize the seriousness of her condition. She looks okay from the front, but the back is horrendous, urine, feces and pus mixing together.

After Mrs. Johnston acquired VRE (vancomycin resistant entero-coccus) in her blood, which a resident said was a deadly organism, an experienced nurse read her chart, telling me indignantly that there was nothing in the chart about her case being hopeless: There was a note by a colorectal resident suggesting whirlpool baths and a divert-ing colostomy, another note mentioning a possible colostomy, but nothing that said that there was almost no chance of this patient leav-ing the hospital alive. The nurse indicated:

> This seems to be what often happens: The doctors don't put down what the nurses—and the doctors—know. They may discuss it verbally, on rounds, but if you look at the chart, there are all sorts of plans for the patient.

The patient's mother came to see her from out of state, and the intensivist on service that week met with the family. He told me that the mother and he had "bonded"—both were deeply religious, and she knew that her daughter would not pull through. When ques-tioned, he reluctantly admitted that the patient's children disagreed. He attributed this to their "emotional immaturity and lack of knowl-edge regarding physiology."

A week later, Mrs. Johnston was still in the unit. Her mother had returned home. When I asked a fellow about her, she responded that the doctors could and did discuss the issues for hours on rounds. A nurse said, of this case and another similar one, that it is the doctors who supposedly make the decisions, but clearly, in these two cases, it is the families. Yet the chances of such patients leaving the SICU are remote. If Mrs. Johnston did manage to get out, she would have to spend a year in a rehabilitation facility. (I wondered, at the time, who was paying and learned later that it was Medicaid.) Said one outspoken resident: "It's been three weeks now, and it's the same old story." "No one wants to get involved, it's so labor–intensive," responded a fellow. "It's labor intensive for the nurses, too," said the resident, "and the orderlies." (In other words, it would be labor intensive to override the children's wishes, possibly involving a court order and much unwelcome publicity. So instead, the nurses had to care for a woman they knew was dying and clean a wound that turned the stomachs of observers.)

A few days later:

> Mrs. Johnston had no major events [her condition did not change]. She's on no sedation and is not responsive. She has persistent fevers and an elevated white count. The family keeps flip-flopping about what to do. Her mother defers to her [the patient's] children; her sister wants to let her go, but her children have decided that they want to do everything, including shocking her. They're sure she'll get better. . . . . Her kidneys are slowly withering away. She seems to be dying, but very very slowly, and her children refuse to give up.

A few days later, the attending said to the fellow: "Siegfried, she's going like this" making a diving motion with his hand. "We're treating the family," he said, obviously disturbed, but just as obviously feeling unable to resolve the issue. "If we treat her all the way," he said, "we could keep her alive for months." It was clear that they were not "treating her all the way," but they were treating her far more than they wished because of the children's insistence. "McDermott [another intensivist] comes on tomorrow," he said. "I'll talk to him. I've done my share."

A nurse observed that the children's eyes became glazed when the doctors attempted to discuss their mother's condition. She felt they were not listening, that they did not *want* to listen. Several nurses reported observing similar reactions from the children, and the nurses were upset about the doctors' unwillingness to make a decision.

Mrs. Johnston's heart finally failed and she died a month after coming to the unit.[16] The children had refused to make her DNR (do not resuscitate) and when she "arrested," they wanted her "shocked." The fellow explained that she was in asystole and that shocking her would not bring her back.[17]

After Mrs. Johnston's death, I learned that several nurses, after overhearing the Johnston children's conversation in their mother's room, were convinced that her pension had influenced their reluctance to allow her to die. The nurses shared their information and surmises with one another, but did not discuss this with the doctors.

I tried cornering the two co-directors of the SICU to learn why, in a case where there was unanimous agreement among the medical staff that further care was futile, a patient was kept alive for almost a month on the insistence of her children. I said that it had been clear that the intensivists had no hope; it was equally clear that no one was going to take the responsibility of moving Mrs. Johnston to comfort care against the wishes of family members. Both directors talked pious generalities.

Was it spinelessness or prudence that kept this dying woman alive (if one can call her condition that) for a month? The laws are uncertain, with some legal decisions supporting the right of families to sustain a patient indefinitely when family members insist this was what that person would have wished. [18] "In today's climate," as one of the directors delicately put it, both doctors and hospitals are terrified of being sued, with the children going to the newspapers with the accusation: "They killed my mom!" This, in fact, was what a cynical resident had told me. He said that poor families are particularly litigious, and poor neighborhoods are filled with lawyers suggesting that, when someone dies in a hospital, a lawsuit might be a reasonable and profitable course of action. Of the Johnston children's insistence on holding out for a miracle, he said, "It's a cultural thing."

End-of-life decisions appeared to be more problematic and time-consuming among African American families.[19] The ICU nurses confirmed this impression. How much of this has to do with distrust, and how much, with a belief in miracles, is impossible to determine. When surveyed about attitudes toward life-sustaining technology by Blackhall et al. (1999), African American respondents gave contradictory responses. Although they indicated that withholding and withdrawing medical care was acceptable under some circumstance, they were more likely than three other groups surveyed[20] to *personally* want to be kept alive by life support. Not only did the African American respondents distrust doctors, feeling that their motives might be tainted by economic considerations, some indicated that only God—rather than doctors—knew everything, with statements such as, "I would want to be put on a machine and be here as long as possible . . . I believe in a power greater than man . . . a miracle or whatever."

I was surprised to discover that the Midwest medical center had been segregated until the 1960s. Thus, each African American family was likely to have members who recall being confined to basement wards. Such "cultural memories" surely do not promote trust. Annette Dula, who examines the sources of the African American mistrust of the health care system, finds it justified. Nevertheless, she concludes that, although such distrust is warranted, it obscures the real problem "of alarmingly poor health, unequal access to healthcare, poverty, violence, and lack of job and education opportunities."[21]

So far as I could tell, the SICU doctors and nurses were color-blind. They took excellent care of African American, European American, and Asian American patients, and I observed no signs of prejudice. Moreover, the doctors went out of their way to ignore the costs of patient care and who paid the bills, if and when they were paid. They seemed to feel that finances were someone else's job, and that their task was to deliver the best medical care possible. On occasion—for example, when a young intensivist ordered a drug that cost $10,000 for three doses for a terminal patient with metastatic cancer—I wondered if, perhaps, they were too oblivious to costs. This attitude, that all patients, including those for whom there is no hope, deserve every possible effort to prolong their lives, no matter what the cost, seems particularly American. (This will be discussed in more detail in the final chapter.)

"It's Already Paid For"

Naturally, the refusal to accept death is not confined to poor or African American families. I was told about Mr. Israel Schneider, an 85-year-old man in comfortable circumstances, whose legs had become paralyzed after a fall. He went to the OR to have a blood clot removed, then to an observation unit, then to "the floor," back to the OR, and then to the SICU.[22] The patient had contracted pneumonia, which was treated in the unit. He was returned to the floor, his pneumonia worsened, and he returned to the SICU. His wife, to whom he had been married for more than 50 years, did not trust the doctors; she believed that they were experimenting on her husband. Mr. Schnei-

der kept ping-ponging back and forth from the hospital to a rehabilitation facility, with his wife orchestrating his treatment, insisting that
she was going to keep him alive. She maintained that since they had
medical insurance, his care was already "paid for." More than four
months after his fall, following several moves from rehabilitation to
the hospital and back again, the patient finally sustained a cardiac arrest and died.[23] Discussing the case, an intensivist said that he got the
impression that Mr. Schneider, when away from his wife, might have
expressed very different wishes. When any of the intensivists encountered the wife in the hospital, she refused to meet their eyes. (No one
knew whether this avoidance was due to anger, shame, or both.)

On occasion, a family member, living in a distant city, who has been
estranged from a dying patient returns to the bedside and attempts to
reverse an agreed-upon move to comfort care. This attempt may be
successful or, at the very least, postpone an inevitable death. Although
it is impossible to analyze the behavior of people one does not know,
the supposition arises that guilt may be involved in this insistence.
Silvester reports this common phenomenon—where a geographically
distant family member returns to the bedside and attempts to reverse
all the agreed-upon decisions of what should be done for a dying patient—is known among neurosurgeons as "the child from the other
coast";[24] the Auckland intensivists called it "the last plane from Sidney."[25]

Ethical Problems, Principles, and Cases

With the exception of the Dalziel family, I have presented problematic cases rather than the far more frequent occasions in which a patient improves and leaves the unit, or families make the painful decision to allow a terminal patient to die, or ask the intensivist: "What
would you do?" and follow his recommendations.

Nevertheless, I have grave doubts about the principle of delegated
autonomy. As Puri and Weber observe: "An undue emphasis on patient autonomy has been interpreted to mean that the family speaks
for incompetent patient with the same authority that a competent patient does."[26] Should family members be burdened with a decision on
whether to "pull the plug on your brother"? Is this truly "autonomy"
or merely a cruel passing–the buck?

In fact, as Puri and Weber ask: "Are concepts of patient autonomy
enough to solve vexing moral problems?" They cite Callahan who
questions the right of competent but dying patients to demand non-

beneficial life extending treatments.[27] (In other words, did 84-year-old Mr. Bascombe have the "right" to request an "incredibly heroic operation" when it would not give him more time?) Abstract principles such as "autonomy" or "benevolence" are singularly unhelpful when dealing with complex real-life cases involving life and death. A moral calculus in terms of cases or stories rather than principles seems a far more productive route.[28] Discussing cases is an age-old method of grappling with moral problems, from Socrates, to the Bible, to the medieval Catholic Church, to Sigmund Freud.[29] Cases, filled with details and difficulties, are how doctors discuss problems.[30]

"I've Seen Patients Like This Survive"

In the Midwest SICU, where responsibility for patients is shared between surgeons and intensivists, families are frequently confused by conflicting messages from the surgeon and intensivist. A surgeon may tell family members that "he's doing fine" when the intensivists are convinced that a patient's condition is terminal. On rare occasions, however, the surgeon's optimism turns out to have been justified. Here is one such case.

Mr. Rob Carnegie was the man whose surgeon, describing the surgical covenant, said: "I looked at him and said 'I'll take care of you' and that was it." This gravely ill man arrived in the SICU after being operated on for cancer. This was not the patient's first hospitalization; he had undergone a number of previous procedures for various illnesses and complications. The patient had a spot on his lung, which may have been metastatic cancer, as well as peripheral vascular disease, and a medical history that included 30 years as a heavy smoker and 45 years of exposure to asbestos. Almost every intensivist had a turn caring for him, and all expressed despondency. "If he doesn't turn around," said one, "the prognosis is really grim."

The surgeon, however, was adamant; the patient was going to get better, and she refused to hear any talk about discontinuing heroic care. She insisted that she be the only person to discuss the patient's condition with his family. "She's one of those it's-my-way-or-the-highway surgeons," commented a nurse. An attending described a public scene she had made in the unit: After he asked if she had told the family that Mr. Carnegie's cancer was possibly metastatic, she had exploded, "screaming" that the intensivists were a bunch of incompetent murderers.

Despite a rocky course, and skepticism on the part of the intensivists, Mr. Carnegie did leave the SICU nine weeks after his arrival, and was eventually discharged from the hospital. He had possible metastatic cancer, but he survived. The surgeon told me that after he left the unit, he asked her: "Is there light at the end of the tunnel?" and she responded, "Yes." She then asked him, "Did you want me to keep you alive?" and he replied, "Yes."

"Every time I see her, she mentions Mr. Carnegie," remarked the co-director of the SICU.

Surgeons, then, can against all likelihood win their battle with the Grim Reaper. I do not know what the odds were for Mr. Carnegie's survival, but I suspect they were slender. Let me "guesstimate" that the odds were approximately 96 percent against this patient leaving the hospital.[31] Surgeons are trained to battle against death and fate. When cases are discussed at the surgical M & Ms, surgeons are never castigated by their colleagues for fighting to the patient's last gasp; they are chided for what they did wrong, or what they did *not* do. The problem is that if a patient has a 96 percent chance of not surviving, and does indeed endure, 96 other dying patients, with dismal prognoses, will be flogged unnecessarily. "I've seen patients like this get better" is the surgeon's mantra.[32] And indeed, patients like this do get better, as did Mr. Carnegie. But if only 4 out of 100 survive, the other 96 may be subjected to futile operations, drugs, and treatments with a heavy cost in time, money, and suffering. And a heavy cost in public resources: scarce ICU beds, Medicare and Medicaid funds, or health insurance companies who, after paying for the care, raise the rates for patients with similar conditions.

In a discussion of whether limiting intensive care at the end of life would save money, Luce and Rubenfeld discuss rising health costs.[33] They indicate that in 1978 and 1988, 6 percent of Medicare recipients over 65 who died accounted for 28 percent of the costs of the program. Seventy-seven percent of the expenses of those who died occurred in the last year of life, 52 percent of them in the last two months, and 40 percent in the last month. Over 70 percent of the total expenses for those who died occurred when these patients were in the hospital. Despite these statistics, however, the authors conclude that limiting intensive care at the end of life would not save money. They advance a number of reasons why, concluding with the assertion that if there were implicit or explicit rationing of intensive care—as there is in countries with limited health care resources such as New Zealand—"the price of such rationing would be to dash the expectations of patients and sacrifice lives that could be saved or *at least prolonged* through ICU admission" [the italics are mine]. They argue that this process has proved to be politically untenable in the United States. This "political untenableness" seems to me to be the crux of their argument. American patients expect care at the end of life, feel it is their "right," and their expectations are dashed when their lives are not prolonged by costly ICU treatments. Is this a medical argument? Or even an ethical one? Or is it a somewhat tautological insistence that Americans hope for and expect such care and therefore limited community resources must be expended for this political necessity?

Who Cares, How, and about Whom?

The administrative model of each of the three units I studied influenced the care given dying patients. The organization of the unit (semiclosed, open, closed) altered the timing and content of communication with patients' families. The moral economies of surgeons as opposed to those of intensivists affected the way they related to patients and families, as did the scheduling of intensivists.

The Covenant of Care in Texas

In the open Texas SICU, where surgeons made decisions about their own patients, I observed less conflict between attendings than in the Midwest ICU, where patient responsibility was shared between surgeons and intensivists. Family members also appeared less confused, since they did not receive diverging messages from surgeons and intensivists. Although financial constraints were mentioned (the hospital where the unit was located was in serious financial difficulties), the covenantal ethic prevailed, and surgeons did not hasten to withdraw care from a gravely ill patient.

The third-year surgical residents assumed a great deal of responsibility, including conducting end-of-life meetings with families to decide whether to discontinue "heroic" care; at this point the patient was made DNR and sent to the floor to die.

I sat in on four such meetings, one held by the "fellow," another by the trauma surgeon who had not yet fulfilled the fellowship requirements, and two conducted by third-year residents. The residents seemed to me to be as capable as the attendings, giving clear, detailed descriptions, in English rather than medical jargon, of the patient's condition and potential courses of action. One resident, a woman from a nearby Air Force base, was outstanding. Here is a description from my fieldnotes of the meeting she conducted:

> Kelly explained what had happened [a life-threatening emergency the previous day], and that it really was a code, even though they didn't have to squeeze the chest. The most worrisome thing was his mental status, explained Kelly. She used some technical terms, but her tone and body language was so warm and compassionate that the technical terms didn't seem to matter. "Is he brain dead?" asked the wife, and Kelly explained that this was a technical term that had all sorts of criteria that needed to be filled before it was decided that someone was brain dead. But his pupils were not responding to light, which is one of the criteria. . . . The wife began to weep, and Kelly put her hand on the wife's arm in a very warm, consoling fashion. Her face, too, was very sympathetic. The nurse said, "We need to take care of you. My first priority is your husband, but you're my second priority." They asked where his parents were and her parents and who they could call to be with her. It seems some family members had left for Dallas and Chicago. "Give me the numbers and I'll call them long distance if you want," said the nurse.

I was not surprised at the nurse's caring behavior but was delighted to observe it in a woman surgeon.[34]

The Texas surgeons took "deliberate speed" in making end-of-life decisions. Families seemed to be consulted when the odds of survival were extremely poor. When I was studying the unit, a 500-pound patient with complications from a gastric by-pass, which included VRE in his blood, had been in the ICU for 64 days. Although residents seemed doubtful that he would survive, the attendings expressed optimism and I heard no talk about withdrawing care. An attending told the residents that this man's difficulties resulted from having been given a long, and unnecessary, course of antibiotics; the fact that his complications stemmed from his medical care, may have affected the surgeons' reluctance to withdraw treatment.[35] Naturally, ICU prognosis is always uncertain, but in this unit, the operating surgeon's optimistic forecasts prevailed.

When the surgeons did decide that there was little hope of survival, a resident or intensivist would schedule a meeting with the family, whose members were asked what they wished to do. They were allowed to take as much time as they felt they needed to make a decision, which could include sending the patient to a long-term care facility.

I observed no occasions where a family insisted on keeping a dying patient going for weeks or months. I suspect that the outcome was relatively clear by the time families were consulted.

More common were situations such as that of Aurelio Limon, a fifteen-year-old, who was shot while attempting to steal some electronic equipment from a store; his companion brandished a toy gun at a guard, whose bullet went through the patient's head, taking fragments of skull and brain with it. Although the patient showed a few faint signs of life, there was no hope of a meaningful recovery.[36] Before the family conference was held, the fellow posed a hypothetical question: "What happens if his dad says he's worthless, he's always been worthless, pull the plug? What do you do?" When the residents admitted they did not know, the fellow said he would have trouble deciding in such a case, as well. The intensivist declared that the overriding principle, legally and ethically, was: What would the patient want? The nurse then told us that she had discussed the matter several times with the family, and she thought that they were ready to let the patient go.

When the parents arrived, a resident who had been caring for him, the intensivist, and I accompanied them to the conference room:

> The father was a small man in jeans with a limp and a pronounced Hispanic accent. The mother, who said nothing, was small and rather heavy with a round face, resembling that of the patient, and enormous eyes. When they [the medical team] explained the situation, which had already been explained to them before, and asked what their decision was, the father said, "I don't want him to suffer. Let God take him. Let him go to heaven and be happy there." Chuck [the resident] told them what would happen. He wasn't great, I think he's only a second-year orthopod [orthopedic resident], but it was good training for him, and Hunter [the intensivist] filled in the details. Hunter said: "But we haven't heard from his mother, what does she think?" The mother agreed with the decision. (She said something to the father in Spanish, and afterwards, Hunter worried that perhaps she was voicing some objection—he can speak Spanish but has some difficulty understanding it. Chuck said no, she was just asking about the vent coming out.) Hunter told them that he might go immediately, or in a few hours, in which case, he'd be kept in the unit; but it might take as long as a week, in which case he would go to the floor, where they could all spend more time with him than they can here. "He was supposed to be in school," said the father, "but they do what they want." . . . They asked the family if they'd like to see him before the tube was removed or wait until it came out, or watch it come out. . . . I noticed a bit later that a young girl was being led from the room, weeping, by another older person, and after that, there was the sound of loud cries from the room.

The resident went into the room and later I learned that the boy had died.

The choices offered families may have differed from those volunteered in the Midwest SICU. Again from my fieldnotes:

> Miss Lopez, age 82, is not with it. Schultz [the "fellow"] decided to stop sedation and see what her mental condition is then. If she doesn't come back, her family will have to decide upon (1) a long-term care facility, (2) switching from cure to comfort care, or (3) discontinuing care. This will take a few days to play out.

The family was not given the alternative of continuing heroic care in the unit.

Although some Hispanic families exhibited dramatic expressions of grief, with screams, frantic weeping, and wailed exclamations: "My brother, my brother, I want him back!" I observed no insistence on waiting for a miracle. When I mentioned the behavior of the African Americans in the Midwest ICU, one of the intensivists responded that African Americans made up only 7 percent of the population in this city, while they comprised 50 percent of the population in Birmingham, where he had trained. He said that the African American families there did behave differently. First of all, the families in Birmingham did not trust the white doctors. He does not blame them, he said, if he were an African American in Alabama, he would not trust the whites either. And then, he declared, there's that "religious thing": They wait for, hope for, expect miracles. They probably believe that so long as the heart is beating, God can do what He wants to do, and if He wants to provide a miracle, He'll do so.

Let us examine another end-of-life situation: Mr. Angel Careno, age 80, who was found unconscious in a ravine the morning after a family celebration. The surgeons operated, performing an "exploratory laparoscopy," to learn what was wrong, and discovered that the patient had Stage 3 lymphoma.[37] Moreover, his liver exhibited unexplained nodes, and it was possible that the cancer had spread to his bones. I was present as a third-year surgery resident talked with two family members. The previous day, the resident had described the patient's grim prognosis and asked the family members to discuss whether the man would have wanted to be kept alive by artificial means. We had expected a large Hispanic family, but there were only two people present, in their twenties or thirties, children perhaps or grandchildren. They indicated that the patient had told his family that he would not want to be kept alive by artificial means. If his heart stopped, or he stopped breathing, would he have wanted to be "coded," asked the resident, describing the emergency procedures that might be followed, and emphasizing that although these might bring the patient back, it would not alter his prognosis. The two family members listened carefully, discussed the matter in Spanish with two more relatives who had arrived, and then said they did not want to use any extraordinary means. In other words, the family was making the patient DNR. The resident then went and filled out a DNR form, saying to me, "Doctors aren't very good at this." But actually, I thought this third-year surgery resident had done a good job and noted that residents were given far more responsibility here than in the Midwest ICU.

When I arrived in the unit at 7:30 the next morning, I learned that the patient had been transferred to the floor. When I inquired, I was told "Oh yes, he's DNR" as though that automatically shifted a patient out of the unit. The resident announced that he had informed the entire gathered family at midnight that the patient would be transferred to the floor where they would all be able to spend much more time with him. He said they were all very grateful.

In another case, where a man in his 90s had shot himself in the head after receiving a diagnosis of metastatic cancer, a third-year resident and I were prepared to discuss end-of-life issues with his wife. We discovered, however, that his 89-year-old wife was deeply confused and did not seem to have a clear idea of what was going on. When the resident and nurse told her "he has a bullet in his head," she asked, "Oh, did it come from the window?" Later, she declared that his two nephews had dropped him off in a box. When they told her the prognosis was grim, she said she wanted to continue because he always said he wanted to live until he was 105. Every member of the wife's family, telephoned by the patient's nurse, declared himself or herself unable to come in. Finally the resident called an intensivist, who came to the bedside and concluded that although they did not have to stop treatment, they could refuse to escalate it.

When I arrived the following morning, the patient had just died. No family member had come to the hospital, with the exception of one young man who may or may not have been a relative. The nurse was trying to locate a priest to come in (the hospital priest was away on a retreat). The old lady wrote something for the nurse that said, in effect, he killed himself because there was no one there to help.

Later that morning, the wife's brother finally arrived and led her off, telling the nurse that he would try to get a social worker to stay with her. "It's a bummer," said the nurse. "I'm glad he [the brother] didn't stay. I was tempted to say something. It makes me mad!"[38]

In this case, no end-of-life decision was made; the patient died, which was apparently his intention.

Although I observed less conflict in this unit, and less confusion among family members, since they received the same message from all the doctors, it is possible that I missed a great deal. Three weeks of observation is limited, and indeed, the chief, in a comment on my discussion of the differences between the three ICUs I studied, felt that, although I was correct in my description of the covenantal ethic, I underestimated the surgeons' consideration of quality of life issues.[39] He emphasized the difficulty, indeed impossibility, of predicting survival and of predicting what the quality of life would be for those who survived. The example he offered was the morbidly obese patient who had been in the unit for 64 days when I left Texas. The chief reported that after a prolonged stay, this patient did, indeed, leave the unit for a rehabilitation facility; he has lost 100 pounds, said the chief, and is "more functional now than prior to his operation."[40]

1

Intensive Caring
in New Zealand

**The success of intensive care is not to be measured only by the
statistics of survival, as though each death were a medical
failure . . . It is to be measured by the quality of lives preserved
or restored, and by the quality of the dying of those in whose
interests it is to die, and by the quality of the human
relationships in each death.**[1]

—G. R. Dunstan

hen I compared the lower-tech Auckland, New Zealand
ICU with its American counterparts, an attending responded: "It's not technology that makes intensive care
work, it's people who intensively care."

Although resources were scarce in New Zealand, the
people in the Auckland ICU did, indeed, intensively care.
They obviously cared about preserving and restoring lives
and, also, about the quality of the dying and the quality of
the human relationships in each death.

Contrasted with in New Zealand, the American medical
system is characterized by abundance. The United States
has 30.4 ICU beds per 100,000 population, while New
Zealand has 5.3 intensive care beds per 100,000; to put it
another way, one ICU bed per 3289 persons versus one
bed per 18,868 persons. In Auckland the pressure is even
more intense: 4.5 beds per 100,000, or one ICU bed per
22,222 persons.

In the closed medical surgical ICU in Auckland, doctors had formal strategies for dealing with scarce resources. They admitted only those patients with "reversible or potentially reversible life-threatening illness or injury." They also limited treatment. This involved: (a) "admitting with reservations," where it was agreed that the patient would be treated only as long as progress seemed reasonable; (b) deciding ahead of time that not all treatments would be offered to a particular patient, or setting an upper limit on the treatment to be offered; and/ or (c) withdrawing treatments when the doctors believed there was little hope of the patient returning to a meaningful quality of life. These difficult decisions were made by consensus; they were group decisions.

Patient care in the New Zealand unit was the primary responsibility of all the critical care doctors. This contrasts with the Midwest SICU, where the physicians worked as anesthesiologists or surgeons, and spent time conducting basic research, and with the Texas unit, where the intensivists worked as trauma surgeons. All the New Zealand intensivists spent most of their working time in the unit. Three of the six intensivists in the 14-bed unit spent 20 percent of their time on other commitments; the other three were employed full time as clinicians. What this meant was that the doctors had more time than their American counterparts to care for patients and to meet with families; most had few other urgent responsibilities that conflicted with this. Their care included thrice-daily rounds, at 8:00 A.M., 4:00 P.M., and 10:00 P.M. as well as "paper rounds" at noon. Clinical studies were carried out, but no intensivist conducted basic research.

More than one intensivist was always present in the Auckland ICU to help make decisions and deliver patient care. Each was on-service for a day at a time, with a backup intensivist *formally* scheduled to be present to help out. Morning rounds generally had at least three attendings participating: the previous day's intensivist, who was handing over the cases to today's critical care physician, the doctor who was on call that day, and the backup intensivist. Moreover, the intensivists' offices were in the unit. This meant that several additional attendings could be hastily recruited to help make a decision. It also meant that when an intensivist conducted a time-consuming meeting with family members, colleagues were in the unit caring for patients.

The critical care doctors were strict about whom they accepted in the ICU. They guarded their "gatekeeper" prerogative closely; on occasion a surgeon might—by incomplete or misleading information—

slip someone who the intensivists believed to be an inappropriate ICU candidate past the gatekeeper into the unit; such a patient, however, was sent to the ward as rapidly as possible. The intensivists were equally strict about limiting care, shifting patients to comfort care when they felt there was little chance of surviving with a meaningful quality of life.

To give just one example of limitation of care from my fieldnotes:

> The fifth [patient we came to on morning rounds] is a 78-year-old man who was in another ICU for three days. He had diarrhea and vomiting—he suffers from emphysema—and they were treating him for pneumonia. [The intensivist] thinks he may well have vomited and aspirated the vomit. He has multiple organ failure. They decided to take him and see how he does. They won't dialyze him for kidney failure but continue ventilating him, allowing him to demonstrate his "robustness" or his lack thereof. If he continues to "circle the drain" they won't offer him a long ICU stay, they'll let him go.

The intensivists had a strong sense of corporate identity and responsibility. Discussing their relations with administrators and other departments, one man declared: "We hunt as a pack!"

The Auckland critical care doctors seemed more interested in the personal situations of each patient than were their American counterparts. During rounds in the Midwest ICU, the resident who presented a case would sketch the "social history" at the end. This seemed to be a somewhat mechanical recitation that could, when time was short, be skipped. The focus of attention was what was wrong with the patient's body and how it could be fixed. Personal information was mentioned earlier in an Auckland resident's recitation it was one of the factors they were expected to discuss—and intensivists often questioned residents and nurses about a patient's family situation: "He lives alone, this guy?" [when told patient was married] "Somebody spoke to his wife?" or "Does the family know how sick she is?" It was clear that speaking to the family was considered an essential part of the intensivist's job, and residents were tutored in the importance of such communication.

The doctors interacted more with patients, as well. Almost all the Auckland patients were awake, and the intensivists would chat with them, ask them how they felt, and, if a patient reached out, clasp that person's hand. They would discuss patients' condition with them: "I know you're tired of us. You're getting better but your lungs are too stiff, you have to stay with us until you can breathe better" or "A bit of light happening at the end of the tunnel. It's taking a long time, but you're getting there." One of the attendings, a woman, would talk to older patients in a tender, daughterly tone: "I'm going to have a look at your tummy, but I'm not going to touch it." One man would joke with patients and family members:

> The patient held out his hand and [the intensivist] took it. . . . He held out his hand again and made it clear he wanted the nurse. "I don't blame you, she's much prettier than I am," said [the intensivist], and the nurse blushed deeply.

This hirsute intensivist, dressed in a blue scrub suit and rubber flip-flop sandals, spent much of his time patrolling the unit, checking the condition of each patient, fixing lines, and performing whatever small procedure was necessary. Every morning before rounds began, he would swing through the two wards checking patients; he was a favorite among patients and families, who would ask for "the hairy doctor."

The Auckland consensual model is influenced by New Zealand values: I was told that egalitarianism and consensus are part of New Zealand's heritage. Star-quality was never mentioned, and I learned that standing out from the group is discouraged. Attendings and nurses quoted a New Zealand saying: "Tall poppies get cut down," and seemed amused when I told them that in the United States, "tall poppies" get appointed chiefs of service. Thus, the location of the New Zealand intensivists' offices, the schedules of the intensivists, and the priority given to consensus, facilitated group decision making at the end-of-life meetings. No one had to make a difficult decision on his or her own; no one was forced to "play God."

The leaderless consensual model was also influenced by the history of this ICU. The intensivists were reacting against the dictatorial practices of the Scottish physician who had founded the unit—and established intensive care as a specialty in New Zealand. (One doctor related how, when he was a resident—the unit took children in those days who would wander around the ICU connected to IVs that trailed behind them—he taught one very young child to give a Nazi salute each time she passed the director!) When the director retired in 1983, the others resolved never to work like that again or work with anyone like that. One intensivist, who had been trained by the critical care autocrat, leaving to conduct research and returning in 1985, introduced the notion of consensus. This intensivist acted as the spark, generating a host of dazzling ideas and suggestions. A colleague provided the fuel, proposing practical ways to implement consensus in decision making, policy development, and documentation. (The second man possessed the rare quality defined by the poet Keats, "negative capability"—a remarkable ability to shut out competing stimuli and concentrate *totally* on the matter at hand.)

Achieving consensus was not necessarily effortless. Although I was on occasion asked to leave the room when the intensivists discussed contentious and/or sensitive issues, it was obvious that consensus took a great deal of time and energy. Consensus involved agreement not only on what to do with each patient, but also on what drugs to be used for various conditions. (This was in contrast to the Midwest unit, where each intensivist had favorite medications he frequently ordered—even when the official policy was to hold off on a particularly expensive drug.)

Consensus was apparently easier in the earlier years of the Auckland ICU, when there were only four critical care doctors; with six, the meetings were longer, and the disagreements, on occasion, more vehement. Deciding to shift a patient from heroic to comfort care took time, sometimes several days, and much discussion, which could grow heated. The intensivists varied, some being swift to suggest discontinuing aggressive care, others taking far longer to agree to such a plan. The idea man, whom I felt would be a "tall poppy" in any other venue, apparently used his intelligence, strength of character, and influence to facilitate consensus. His colleague implemented consensus in his own fashion, methodically collecting everyone's ideas, writing multiple drafts of potential courses of action, and stubbornly keeping the group going until agreement was achieved. Each person's contributions acted as a kind of "glue" to hold the unit together.[2] However, the closeness of the intensivists, the fact that they spent so much time together, magnified the intensity of the disagreements that did erupt. Just as family fights can be more ferocious, the conflict among the intensivists could become devastatingly painful. I was told of disagreements where the unit threatened to split asunder, with threats of someone leaving or being asked to leave. But so far, the hard-won consensus prevailed.[3] (A new hospital was under construction, with a larger ICU planned; adding intensivists to the staff might make consensus even more difficult and time-consuming.)

The New Zealand ethos of egalitarianism extended beyond the relationship between intensivists: I observed a less hierarchical relationship between doctors and nurses than in the United States. The doctors seemed to really listen to nurses and respect their opinions.

During rounds, after a resident summarized each patient's condition, an attending would ask the nurse: "Do you have anything to add?" This was not a pro forma question; the intensivists appeared genuinely interested in nurses' evaluations of patients' physical and emotional states as well as their family situations. Nurses, residents, and intensivists were on a first-name basis.[4]

The 1-to-1 nurse–patient ratio in the New Zealand ICU meant that nurses learned a great deal about the patient and visiting family during 12 hours of caring for that person.[5] The fact that most patients were awake facilitated communication. Naturally, it was the 1-to-1 ratio that reduced the risk of self-injury, making it less dangerous to keep patients awake.[6] The staff was proud of the fact that, in contrast to American units, the Auckland ICU patients never developed pressure sores; a nurse was always present to tilt the bed at various extreme angles so that the patient did not rest in the same position long enough to develop sores. A very sick patient who needed complex management might be assigned two nurses. In addition, each of the two ICU wards had a "runner," a nurse formally scheduled to help out when another pair of hands was needed. (In contrast, the two American ICUs had a 1-to-2 nurse–patient ratio, although very sick patients might be assigned a single nurse. Aides and respiratory technicians assisted the American nurses.) Aides and respiratory techs were not in evidence in the Auckland ICU, where each nurse had sole responsibility for the patient. I was told that this policy was intentional; the nurse did *everything* for the patient. An intensivist declared that this improved care and promoted bonding between nurse, patient, and family. When family conferences were scheduled, the nurse attended and often remained to answer questions and comfort family members after the intensivist had left the room.

Respect and Responsibility

ICU nursing supervisors and intensivists carried out what appeared to be an organized effort to encourage nurses to acquire new skills and grow professionally.[7] In addition, a peer support group met regularly, where nurses could discuss upsetting incidents and interactions. There was a separate support group for new nurses to help integrate them into the unit. Although other departments in the hospital and throughout New Zealand, suffered from a nurse shortage, the Auckland ICU had a waiting list of nurses who wanted to work there.

The nurses in the Auckland ICU were accorded respect and responsibility. Many American doctors and supervisors seem to disrespect nurses, giving them little true responsibility and few opportunities to grow professionally. Yes, an American nurse can attend graduate school,[8] but that is not quite the same as *opportunities to learn and grow on the job*. To give just one example of disrespect among a multitude in my fieldnotes: in the Midwest ICU, a fellow could—and frequently did— enter the rooms of patients placed on isolation status, neglecting to glove and gown, ignoring the cautions of a highly experienced nurse.[9] Such behavior was overlooked by superiors; he was a "star," she was a nurse, and their status on the food chain was unmistakable.

I suspect that American doctors, with few exceptions, disrespect nonphysicians. This is deeply below the level of consciousness, and most doctors are unaware of their gut feelings of superiority, even if it is only manifested in terms of compassion for those who know less. (Patients and families, however, are acutely sensitive to this, which is why many family members prefer to ask nurses what is going on.)[10] If one questioned an American doctor, he (and often even she) would declare, and believe this declaration, that he surely respects nurses— rather like the old Mike Nichols–Elaine May skit, where the teenaged boy, trying to get a girl to go "all the way" assures her, "I respect you like crazy!" Consider the multisite study to improve care at the end of life, where highly trained nurses reported patient prognoses to doctors, who then ignored these reports.[11] This behavior did not surprise me, but the project's lack of success seems to have astonished the investigators, who so far as I could tell, did not attribute this failure to doctors' inability to listen to what nurses tell them. I suspect the investigators *scientific* credentials were impeccable, but their *social* knowledge of doctor–nurse interaction left something to be desired.[12] Fortunately, this disrespect is not universal in the United States: I spent a day in a midwestern cardiac care ICU, where the nurses were given a great deal of responsibility, being allowed to write orders for patients, which were then carried out and subsequently signed by the cardiac surgeons. A physician friend with a relative in the unit told me how impressed he was when he heard a cardiac surgeon teaching the nurses: The man was teaching them how to think and exercise judgment, telling them what to look for and how to evaluate what they saw, rather than how to carry out procedures by rote—which is how I have observed most American nurses in most sites being taught. The nurses reported that they had *no* nurse turnover in that unit.

Although cardiac intensive care surely differs from surgical care, respect and responsibility are either accorded nurses or not—and when they are absent, nurses vote with their feet.

New Zealand nurses accompany patients who wish to die at home and care for them there. I was told that the Auckland unit has one or two such cases a year; two nurses, or a nurse and a doctor, go home with the patient; the nurses stay with the patient until he or she dies.[13] An Auckland intensivist described accompanying a man who had an inoperable tumor in his throat. There were about 30 people in the room, and although the patient, who had been given a great deal of morphine, was gasping for air, the family was wonderful. Several, were musicians, and as the man died, they were on the side, with guitars, playing his favorite music. I said I found it impossible to imagine something like this occurring in the United States; among other barriers, sending two nurses would mean that four ICU patients were without a nurse. The Auckland intensivist responded that it is a bit hard in their unit when two nurses are gone, but it was clear that he felt this was well worth it.

The nurses and intensivists participate in a moral economy, a system of affect-saturated values, where considering "the quality of the dying of those in whose interests it is to die, and . . . the quality of the human relationships in each death" is perceived as part of their *professional role*. Although some palliative care specialists in the United States share these values, this moral economy does not flourish in most high-tech, scientifically oriented, financially beleaguered American tertiary care centers.

When I e-mailed a senior Auckland ICU nurse asking her if indeed they had a less hierarchical relation between nurses and intensivists, she responded:

> Over the past 10 to 15 years I have noted a continual change in medical staff's attitudes to nurses. I think this has occurred due to:
>
> a) Nursing lifting their education standard and therefore nurses having a better understanding of medical management and a better medical language to interact with medical staff;
>
> b) Even more powerfully, nurses undertaking clinical audit in the form of follow-up and the nurses having the communication skills to address positive and negative comment directly with medical staff. This feedback from patients and the next-of-kin has lifted their communication skills.
>
> c) Nurses are more skilled in being assertive and not accepting crappy, egotistical, prima donna behavior. They will make a time that is suit-

able to the doctor and themselves and address the issue. It then becomes apparent to them [the doctors] (after a couple of these sessions) that they cannot get away with it. Some [doctors] of course do not require it.

The "clinical audit" conducted by nurses did indeed help level the relationship between nurses and intensivists. This feedback loop from the nurses' Bereavement Follow-up Service will be discussed in a subsequent chapter.

Sociability between doctors and nurses was encouraged by the "geography" of the Auckland unit.[14] The Midwest SICU contained a series of widely separated rooms where various groups tended to congregate and eat their lunches: an anteroom adjacent to the nurses' dressing room, with a refrigerator, electric coffee maker, and microwave oven, used primarily by the nurses; another room, with eating facilities, where the technicians gathered; a small room where the residents generally relaxed and ate meals brought from the cafeteria; and an office in the rear of the unit, holding computers for each fellow, and a private room for the attending on service that week, where the fellows and on-service attending tended to spend time when not caring for patients. Although almost everyone used the coffee machine in the "nurses' room," staff members generally ate with their peers. Naturally, while people ate, they chatted, exchanging social, personal, and professional information. Although this segregation was probably unintentional, it sustained a social division between the professional groupings. In contrast, the Auckland ICU held a centrally located "tearoom," where intensivists, residents, nurses, and orderlies congregated. The tearoom contained two refrigerators, one of which was stocked daily with milk by a hospital employee; tea bags, sugar, instant and ground coffee, and a machine that dispensed boiling water; bread, Marmite (a spread beloved by Britons), and a toaster oven; a microwave; a dishwasher; several copies of the day's newspapers; a table where people sat to eat lunches; and rows of comfortable chairs where ICU staff members sat, ate, chatted, and exchanged information. There was also a bulletin board with notices and information of interest to everyone.

"People Who Intensively Care"

One day, an intensivist telephoned me at my apartment, located around the corner from the hospital, to make sure I did not miss the second of four end-of-life conferences with the family of one woman.

After the conference, the patient's nurse, who had returned to the bedside, asked me to give a message to the doctor: "You were *wonderful!* Thank you!" That day, as I ate my lunch in the tearoom, a senior nurse quietly suggested that I give my medical history to an intensivist; she said that in case anything happened, it might be good to know. A secretary sitting with us, who knew I was nervous about driving on the "wrong" side of the road in my newly rented automobile, inquired: "Is that because she just got the car?" The nurse nodded and smiled. As I typed my fieldnotes that afternoon, the nurse's inquiry, plus the thoughtfulness of the intensivists, all of whom went out of their way to notify me when they held end-of-life meetings, in addition to several weeks of observing the way in which intensivists talked of and behaved toward patients and family members, coalesced into a pattern. I realized that in this ICU, everyone exhibited a tremendous respect for others: for patients, families, co-workers, the visiting anthropologist. This respect was *not* evident among the doctors in the Midwest medical center, where professional esteem was focused primarily on "medicine" and "science." The doctors did not exhibit disrespect, but respect and consideration were not identified as an integral part of their professional role.

I cannot estimate how much of this kindness and respect was a New Zealand characteristic and how much was specific to the Auckland ICU. National differences in behavior between New Zealand and the United States were evident. People were more informal in New Zealand; I observed barefoot men entering the hospital wearing shorts. No one seemed surprised by their costume. Kidnappings and crimes of violence were rare; when such a crime occurred, it generated newspaper headlines for days. I was told that the Auckland ICU received a victim of a serious crime of violence every year or so—as opposed to the American units, where patients suffering from gunshot wounds, knifings, and bludgeonings arrived almost every week.[15] (The Midwest unit did not put the names of victims of violence on their doors; on one occasion, a friend of the perpetrator had attempted to enter the unit and finish the job.) New Zealand is apparently a less violent society, and a less litigious one—they have far fewer malpractice suits against doctors. The unit did receive one spectacular case of violence while I was conducting research: after being accused of child abuse, a Samoan man had attacked his two Maori sisters-in-law with a sledgehammer; then, sitting in his car (which he had set on fire), he stabbed himself in the heart. He survived, as did his pregnant sister-in-law, who gave birth after the attack. For a short time, both were in the unit, until the doctors, fearing some sort of retaliation from the victims' family, managed to get the attacker transferred to another hospital.

"It's Not Technology that Makes Intensive Care Work"

Discussing ethical dilemmas in geriatric medicine, Kaufman observes that: "The technological imperative in medicine—to order ever more diagnostic tests, to perform procedures, to intervene with respirators or feeding tubes to prolong life or stave off death—is an important variable in contemporary medical practice"[16] She points out that this imperative determines thought and action, confining choice to black-and-white terms and forcing doctors to think of good, adequate, appropriate medical care as embodied in maximum intervention.

The technological imperative appeared less urgent in New Zealand. Although the intensivists said that they had access to any technology they felt absolutely necessary, the Auckland unit was conspicuously lower-tech than the American ICUs. There were no computers in each room, on which doctors could access information about that patient—just one, for each of the two ICU wings (plus somewhat antique computers in each intensivist's office); large paper charts were used instead. In place of a computer setup that displayed X rays, the actual X rays were examined by residents and intensivists, who pulled out large screens holding the films.[17] Moreover, the intensivists administered far fewer antibiotics than their American counterparts. When patients acquired a dangerous drug-resistant organism, patients would be isolated to contain it, rather than given stronger antibiotics. (Naturally, such containment is easier, with a 1-to-1 nurse–patient ratio.) I was told that the dreaded VRE—Vancomycin-resistant enterococcus—was rare in New Zealand since Vancomycin was infrequently administered; only six cases in the entire country had been documented. Some of these differences in technology may have been affected by a shortage of funds, as the New Zealand medical system was desperately short of money. But a philosophical difference existed, as well. Several doctors made pointed "jokes" about Americans attempting to solve problems by throwing money at them; these remarks seemed to be more a moral critique than a product of envy. Because economies are effected in the Auckland ICU by limiting care to those judged able to benefit by such care—as opposed to the American practice of saving money by limiting those who care for ICU patients—the number of patients whose dying is prolonged by the technological imperative is curtailed.

The New Zealand ICU was notable, then, not for its technology, which was somewhat dated when compared with the state-of-the-art units I studied in the Midwest and Texas. But the intensity of caring was remarkable—and heartening. I recalled the Midwest fellow who had said: "One of the problems is that there's no model for anything else. If there were a model for another way of doing things, then we could say, 'Well, this way is better'" (Chapter 2). At the time, I had not known what to tell her, but it did seem that, in many ways—from the curtailed hours of registrars (residents), to the 1-on-1 nurse–patient ratio, to the compassion and concern shown by doctors and nurses—the Auckland way *was* better. Perhaps I'm being naïve, perhaps state-of-the-art technology, with a primary focus on evidence-based medicine, increases the odds of a patient recovering and leaving the ICU. Outcome statistics can be unreliable, since it is difficult, perhaps impossible, to evaluate and compare the population of patients admitted to various ICUs. In the end, all I can say is that should I need intensive care, I would prefer being sent to the Auckland unit.

Intensive caring was demonstrated in a variety of settings, not only in the relationships between Auckland intensivists, nurses, patients, and family members. The doctors spent time and energy *preventing* situations that brought patients to the ICU. I was told of three successful campaigns they initiated.

First, they used newspaper and television publicity to lobby for median dividers on the major highways around Auckland that, when installed, significantly reduced the number of serious traffic accidents.

They instigated the *second* campaign to increase the effectiveness of the ambulance service when dealing with trauma. The intensivists conducted studies analyzing all the trauma cases: measuring how long it took to transport patients to an emergency room and documenting what happened when serious cases were brought to the nearest ER rather than to a first-class trauma center, being transferred only when it was decided that the prognosis was grave. After working out indexes to determine the seriousness of the injury, with about 95 percent predictability, one man constructed tables and used these to lobby officials. The campaign was successful, and the Auckland ambulance services changed their practices to include assessing the seriousness of trauma injuries on the spot using the indexes, bringing serious cases directly to one of the two major trauma centers, notifying the ER ahead of time, and deciding which center to go to by the time of day and ease of getting there, rather than by geographic proximity.[18]

The *third* campaign was initiated to cut the recreational use of GHB (the street name of this is Fantasy).[19] The youngest intensivist, a handsome, charming, personable man, went on television, discussing the difficulties associated with use of this drug and describing the patients who died, and those who had vomited, aspirated, and nearly died. Another doctor put the information together and lobbied; eventually, the drug was put on the prohibited list with strong penalties for making or selling it.

Although some American associations of trauma surgeons have lobbied to reduce dangerous conditions, I know of no situations where individuals from one ICU did so. (Naturally, such campaigns are far easier to conduct in a small country with a centralized government, where a state-by-state effort does not have to be conducted.)

Going Gentle into that Good Night

Death in Auckland

"Completion for the Family and for the Nurse"

n the mid-1990s, the Auckland ICU initiated a Survivor's Follow-up Service to interview patients who had been in the unit. These interviews were originally designed as a quantitative "audit" of the effectiveness of ICU systems, service, and patients' current health status. The feelings of former patients, however, became increasingly important to the nurse-interviewers and the doctors who received their reports. A Bereavement Follow-up Service was then initiated.

In 2002, the Bereavement Follow-up Service had been operating for seven years. The nurses' reports, which were circulated in the unit, described not only how the families felt and how they reacted to what the doctors had said and done, but also how these interviews had affected the nurses and their work.

An intensivist introduced me to a nurse who had worked on the Bereavement Team for seven years. When asked whether she found this work depressing, she responded: "Oh no!" She reported that the nurses take turns doing bereavement work for two months each year. They telephone next of kin four to six weeks after a patient's demise to inquire about the care their loved one received, how they themselves were treated, and about their present emotional condition. She was recently on the phone with a woman for 80 minutes. "These people pour out their hearts," she declared, "they have so much they want to say, and it may be easier on the telephone when they don't meet the person they're speaking to. Often their families don't want to hear it, all about the person who died. They tell the most intimate details." This woman found this work so rewarding that she had recently acquired a diploma in counseling, to work with bereaved families.

I was told that the nurses are paid for their time on the service. Nurses in the Midwest SICU had formed a Bereavement Committee, where they discussed how they dealt with bereaved families and drafted letters of condolence, which were sent to next of kin; these efforts, however, were voluntary. The difference between paying and not paying nurses to communicate with bereaved families indicates the importance given to this work by New Zealand versus American administrators and intensivists. The nurse-interviewers of the Auckland Survivors' Follow-up Team are also paid for the time they spend contacting former patients. In the Midwest medical center, on the other hand, professional interviewers contact a selected sample of survivors to question them about their stay. The distinction between the two practices underlines the difference between intensive caring and merchandising.

I attended an annual day-long meeting of the Bereavement Team, attended by six nurses and a senior Clinical Nurse Consultant. I was told that the team members had been selected for their nursing experience and "people skills." They were an impressive group: intelligent, caring, dedicated. The meeting began with a joint breakfast at a local coffee shop; we then moved to a conference room at a nearby lodge (where cancer patients receiving treatment could stay).

The first order of business was to run through the complaints by family members, discussing how each had been dealt with and what might further improve the way dying patients and their families were treated. It was obvious that every complaint was taken very seriously.

The commitment of the team members was apparent. One woman described how, when she heard that the patient's wife she had telephoned was in the hospital, she had left her phone number so that the woman could call her when she got out.

Various people came to talk to the team during the day. A nurse-coordinator discussed what happens to bodies after a patient dies. She said that some families want to take the bodies home, describing how she fulfills these requests; Maori patients want body parts as well, placentas, gall bladders, and so forth. A team member explained that the Maori, the original inhabitants of New Zealand, are often called "people of the land" but that the actual translation is "people who are the land," and the idea is that everything should be returned to the land. The nurses reported that Maori families frequently would come for the body with just a car; there had been automobile accidents and difficulties when a dead body was found, however, so the present rule was that the body had to be in a "suitable container"—a box or body bag. But one family wanted the body bag unzipped so that the family member could see everything on his journey home! The nurses were distressed when they learned that nurses at a neighboring hospital turn dead patients over to the coroner to deal with. "Dealing with death properly," said one, "gives completion for the family *and* for the nurse. If they're all right, you're all right."

I was told that if someone dies, the space must be blessed before anyone else can be put there. "Who blesses it?" I asked, and was told that anyone who is "spiritually evolved" can do this.[1]

Later, two representatives of a widows and widower's group discussed their organization; the nurses took leaflets to distribute to interested next of kin. Then a social worker spoke of her work with trauma patients and their families; she described this as "trying to normalize the human condition." Two team members reported on a lecture they had attended on death and dying; they were enthusiastic about the American lecturer, telling how he had declared that one's relationship with a loved person does not end when they die, they live on in your heart and influence your life: "He's like a good Jewish father!" said one woman.

The team members keep diaries describing each phone call (in addition to filling out a form with information that is then quantified), and each woman read out portions of her diary. A nurse read a touching poem written by a husband about the death of his wife; he had given permission for the nurses to use the poem in their work. One woman, who was new to the group, told how nervous she was before making a phone call. "Oh, you're always nervous," the others assured her. "You just become familiar with the discomfort grief brings you," said one. The nurses seemed to feel that anyone insensitive enough *not* to feel nervous would be an unsuitable candidate for the team.

One team member described a Bereavement Meeting some time after the death of a family member. Intensivists hold these meetings when the next of kin cannot seem to move on with their grieving and "get stuck" with the same concerns echoed over and over. The intensivist who conducted the meeting did a great deal of research beforehand to find out about the person who died, telephoning the patient's general practitioner to find out more about him and his health. The nurses said that some of the intensivists prepare with great care for these meetings: "There's nothing we ask for that they don't do," she reported. "They say, 'We can do that!'"

I was impressed by the commitment and caring of these nurses—and by the commitment of the nurse-administrators and intensivists to this work. The findings were posted on the tearoom bulletin board; in addition, the nurses informed each intensivist directly about behavior that had disturbed next of kin. This had apparently modified many of the practices in the unit, cutting the number of complaints from 51 percent in 1995, when the Bereavement Follow-up Service was initiated, to 13 percent in 2001. As the nurse who e-mailed me indicated, the Follow-up Service also altered the relationship between nurses and intensivists: The nurses were more outspoken when they observed objectionable behavior from doctors, and the intensivists listened to nurses more carefully. And nurses, residents, and intensivists began to focus more attentively on alleviating the suffering of the families of dying patients.

"That's What We Do Here"

I attended a Bereavement Meeting scheduled by one intensivist. The nurse who had arranged it asked the family if I could attend, and they assented. The intensivist, who usually wore leather sandals, had changed into proper shoes for the conference; this seemed a lovely gesture, symbolic of respect for the occasion, for grief, for death.

A woman and her teenaged daughter had questions about how their husband and father had died. This 52-year-old man had been surfboarding at a company function, suffered a stroke, and fell off the surfboard, inhaling a large quantity of water. The wife's primary question was: If things had been done differently—if the ambulance had come faster, if he had been given different treatment immediately—could he have survived? The intensivist went through the man's medical chart, showing the wife and daughter all the notations and explaining each, telling them about stroke, using a large picture of the brain that the nurse brought in. He showed where the blockage was, what was done for the patient, and how no more could be done. He read them the chart summary and autopsy report, explaining everything with great patience and clarity. The intensivist, a quiet, reserved man, left a great deal of time for the wife and daughter to formulate and pose questions. "Could the blockage come from somewhere else?" "The only other place it could possibly have come from was his heart, and his heart was given to someone else, and is working well," responded the intensivist, "so that's unlikely." (The fact that someone had his heart and it was working well seemed to comfort the wife.) "Did he suffer? Could something have been done differently?" The intensivist assured her that he did not suffer and that once he had that kind of stroke there was nothing that could be done because part of his brain was blocked. He showed them which artery was blocked, and how the brain on that side swelled out, pushing into the other side, and pushing the cord that controls movement between them. "Would you like copies of these?" the intensivist asked, about the chart summary and autopsy report. They were not sure, but decided to take them, even if they did not keep them. As he left the room to copy them, the intensivist said, "Perhaps you'll think of more questions while I'm gone. Did I answer all the questions in your letter?" It had been a busy, stressful day, but the intensivist behaved as though he had all the time in the world, leaving many spaces where the wife and daughter could think of and pose questions. When they left, the wife and daughter appeared disburdened.

I told the intensivist that I did not remember a doctor speaking so little and allowing so much time for patients to talk: In my experience, doctors usually talk and patients listen. "That's what we do here," he responded quietly.

Who Decides?

> And you, my father, there on that sad height,
> Curse, bless, me now with your fierce tears, I pray.
> Do not go gentle into that good night,
> Rage, rage against the dying of the light.
> —Dylan Thomas

Families were not asked to make end-of-life decisions in the Auckland ICU. In this unit, as well as three other New Zealand units visited briefly, the decision to withdraw therapy and shift to comfort care was made by the doctors, who then invited the family members to agree. "There's always a subtext if you give them [the family] the decisions," said one intensivist: "Do you love this person? How can someone say 'I want this person to die'?"

Is the poet who urges his father to "rage against the dying of the light" the best person to decide how that father should die? As I learned in the Midwest SICU, asking family members "what would your father have wanted?" does not always elicit a decision that the patient, if able to speak, would have chosen—or one that is necessarily in the best interests of the patient.

Death may well be a more tolerable subject for discussion in New Zealand.[2] Although it is becoming more acceptable in the United States, we still find it difficult to discuss dying, to plan for it, and to talk about Do Not Resuscitate (DNR) orders. Doctors find this just as difficult as laypersons. Death is one of the last frontiers. Comparative strangers will tell one in distressing detail about their sex lives. But death—and money—are prohibited subjects. The anxiety of the Midwest doctors, during recorded end-of-life discussions with families, was displayed in their use of medical terms that most laypersons would have difficulty understanding, their complex and torturous phraseology, and in their rapid and apprehensive filling of any silences that might break out.

The New Zealand doctors presented decisions to move from cure to comfort care as unequivocal *medical* judgments, emphasizing that neither they nor family members were killing the patient, it was the injury or disease that was responsible for the death. They spoke in terms of "not prolonging the dying," rather than asking for a family decision on whether or not to allow the patient to die.

Intensivists would usually hold several meetings with families. Here are my fieldnotes about one such discussion in New Zealand:

[The intensivist] went through her entire history, and then said that she was not improving, but just going up and down, and that she was very weak and that there was a strong possibility that she might not ever get out of the hospital. She might meet with some catastrophic event and if she does she probably won't survive. He said this in several ways, so that it was impossible for them *not* to understand. He indicated that she might survive but that there was a strong possibility that she would not, that she was very very weak, and that she couldn't survive a catastrophic event. "Is there anything we can do?" her husband asked. "Take care of yourselves," said [the intensivist]. "If she gets out, she will need a lot of support from you." The husband thanked [the intensivist] twice for being so honest.

A doctor at one New Zealand ICU said that in the first meeting, the intensivist sets the scene: this person is very sick, this is what we hope will happen, but it may not happen, and then we'll have to make some decisions. "You've got to get trust," he said, "You work with them and if there are difficulties, you plan another meeting." With this doctor, as with another at an ICU I visited briefly, the question "what if the family never agrees," seemed to make no sense. Both men apparently felt that if one held several meetings, spoke honestly and openly, and gained trust, the families always came around. "When there are difficulties," said one, "you have to ask [family members] 'Are you doing this because it's the best thing for them?' Often they have to go home and think about it for twenty-four hours before they come back and say 'You're right!'"

A meeting in the Auckland ICU might last as long as 50 minutes; the intensivists knew there were colleagues in the unit caring for patients and had few competing responsibilities to draw them away. I was impressed, during these meetings, by how much time the doctors gave families to speak. The New Zealand doctors *truly listened* to what family members said.

Attending these meetings, I longed for some sort of instrument to calculate who spoke and for how long. The equilibrium between the speech of doctors and of family members seemed far more balanced than in the United States where, in the end-of-life interviews recorded by our project, the doctors did almost all the talking. The New Zealand doctors did not seem afraid of silence. When silence broke out in an American meeting, the doctor would hasten to fill the void with words. The New Zealand doctors asked questions, and then waited, allowing family members to formulate what they wished to ask. The doctors gave no nonverbal signs of impatience and kept meetings going until the family displayed both verbal and nonverbal signs of agreeing with the decision and being, at least somewhat, at peace with it. Each intensivist had a different style, but each seemed to display the same patience and lack of haste during these interviews. Each used a minimum of medical phraseology.

During one such meeting, a daughter asked, "What if we didn't agree?" "We'd meet again, and then meet again, until you understood and agreed," said the doctor, adding, "most families are pretty reasonable and know that the person would not want to survive like that." The family (which included the patients' four children and the wife of one son) seemed grief-stricken but at peace with the decision by the end of this particular meeting. My fieldnotes observed:

> But all of this took *time*, and it seemed to me that the least sign of impatience from [the intensivist]—like [a Midwest intensivist] wriggling or using his this-is-the-end-of-the-conversation-I'm-a-busy-doctor tone of voice would have changed the atmosphere and effect. . . . As it is, [the Auckland intensivist] kept asking: "Do you have any questions? If you think of any questions later, just contact me. I'll be here, although I'll go home for dinner, I can be easily reached, just tell the nurses and they'll get me."

At a meeting with the same family two days earlier, held by two different intensivists, I noted,

> the doctors did between half and two-thirds of the talking. There were many moments of silence, while they waited for the family to formulate questions or decide what they wanted to do. It was a far more egalitarian relationship, signaled by who had the floor. . . . The conference began at about 2:00 and lasted until 2:35 or so, without the slightest sign of impatience from [either of the two intensivists]. They were utterly *there* for the family and the family could feel it. They listened as well as speaking.

Although they brought up the question, this patient's children were unable to decide whether their mother should be told she was dying. During morning rounds, three intensivists discussed whether they should tell this woman. "How is this handled in the US," I was asked, and I replied that the patients in the Midwest SICU are usually so deeply sedated that the issue does not arise. The doctors discussed whether it was their job to inform this woman that she was dying. Two intensivists said that they, themselves, would prefer not knowing; another, preferred knowing. One declared: "It might make us feel better to tell her, as though we were doing the right thing. But is it our place to make such a decision? It's really something the family should decide." I never heard a discussion of this sort in the Midwest unit, perhaps because the patients were unconscious, perhaps because several intensivists were rarely together in the unit, or perhaps because the doctors did not conceptualize such issues as part of their work. The Auckland doctors clearly felt that the moral realm was *their* responsibility and that they were obliged to do the right thing.

The intensivists quoted an article on withholding and withdrawing life-saving treatment by Grant Gillet, a New Zealand surgeon-ethi-cist.[3] The author argues that when making such decisions, we should not think of life versus death; instead, we must consider a third cate-gory: survival in an unacceptably bad state for the patient concerned. Gillet terms this alternative "the RUB," the Risk of Unacceptable Badness. He notes that a patient who is given a probabilistic chance of surviving may picture a small chance of life versus a black hole—death. Faced with these two choices, many may say, "Well, doctor, go for it, after all any chance is better than none." The real probabilities, however, are different: Survival may mean that the person will be left in an unacceptably bad state. Thus a patient with a severe brain injury may have a 5 percent chance of survival, but if he survives, have only a 10 percent chance of living in a state he would find acceptable and a 90 percent chance of living in a state he would consider unacceptably bad. Although the RUB is not a concept that should explicitly be used with patients and relatives, it should inform clinicians' ethical deci-sions. The role of the family, then, is to tell the decision makers, first, what they know the person to have been like and—less significantly because of possible conflicts of interest or other factors—what rela-tives think the patient would have wanted. Gillet concludes that con-sidering this third alternative does not make life-and-death decision making easier and may even make it harder. But it does make it more responsive to "the hopes and fears of any person faced with the mortal perils that often wait at a hospital door."

This point of view, in direct opposition to the surgical covenant viewing death as the supreme enemy, was prevalent among the New Zealand intensivists. Death, then, was not necessarily a defeat, but a tragic and inevitable necessity, when counterposed against a more agonizing outcome.

"The Quality of the Dying of Those Whose Interest It Is to Die"

Let us examine the death of three patients in the Auckland ICU. Al-though every loss of a loved family member is tragic, two of these cases were particularly difficult because they concerned a young per-son who by all rights should have enjoyed a long and productive life.

The first patient, Mrs. Murray, arrived in the unit on a Tuesday, a day before Miss Kline, the second patient whose death we consider. She died on a Saturday, a day before Miss Kline, as well.

"It's Not Her Time to Go!"

I was printing out a description of my research to be placed on the wall of a little family waiting room,[4] when a call came over the loud-speaker: "Doctor, to West One now please! Doctor, to West One now please!" An intensivist ran toward Room #1 in the West Ward with me following. A new patient had arrived, after having collapsed on the ward, and doctors, nurses, and residents were crowded around the bed. A resident rhythmically pressed a rubber bag to assist her breathing, while three intensivists, two nurses, and another resident inserted a tube down her throat that was then attached to the ventilator, inserted lines, connected her to various machines, and moved her from the wheeled bed she had arrived in to the ICU bed. The team worked together with few words. Everyone seemed to know just what he or she should do, and did it.

Mrs. Anne Murray, age 65, had been on the floor when she lapsed into a sudden coma, coughing up blood. She had been diagnosed with cancer of the kidney in a previous hospital, where she had contracted pneumonia, before being transferred to the Auckland University Hospital. An X ray, performed at the bedside, showed the pneumonia, but the doctors thought she might have also suffered a pulmonary embolism.[5] The patient was sent for a CT scan, which diagnosed "a massive pulmonary embolism."[6] Later that morning, the doctors examined the X rays taken at the previous hospital, and by noon they had learned that the patient had cancer in both kidneys, with cancer cells in a lung as well. It was not clear whether kidney cancer had spread to the lung, or whether it was a separate cancer; the patient had been a heavy smoker for many years.

A family conference was scheduled for the following day. Mrs. Murray's husband and her two daughters attended. One daughter, who seemed to be the older of the two, had come from Australia; the second, a small, fine-boned woman, lived in Auckland. The family, the patient's nurse, an intensivist, and I went to the little waiting room. Here is a description from my fieldnotes:

> [The intensivist] began by relating their mother's entire history, then telling them about the cancer in both kidneys and the lungs, and saying that if it were in one kidney, they might think about removing it, but in both kidneys, there was little that could be done. One daughter was very resistant. "She can't die, she's not ready to go!" she kept declaring. "She's a fighter. She'd be so mad!" she kept saying. [The intensivist] sat there with no sign of impa-

tience, not verbal or physical, allowing her to speak, as well as the others, then telling them that they were going to give her 24 hours to see if she rallied; if she rallied, if she could breathe better without help, perhaps, as a best-case scenario, she might be able to leave the ICU and perhaps the hospital, although the cancer had probably spread throughout her body—even though it could not yet be seen on the scans. The daughter kept bargaining for time. "It's not her time to go!" she declared, "You've got to try harder. Can't you remove the kidney?" [The intensivist] said she was in no shape for an operation and that they couldn't remove both kidneys. "Can't you give her more time?" the daughter implored. The husband seemed to understand the situation as apparently did the other daughter, but the one daughter was distraught. "She wants to live!" she insisted. [The intensivist] finally said, "Well I'll leave you to talk things over." "Yes, please do," said the husband.

When I complimented the intensivist on speaking in terms that the family could understand, he responded, "I learned plain English from ['the hairy doctor']."

The patient did not do well that night. A second family conference was scheduled the following morning. Mr. Murray, his two daughters, and the husband of the younger daughter attended. Although the intensivist spoke of a "primary," which I am not sure the family understood, he spoke English most of the time. The daughter from Australia asked excellent questions. The younger daughter, although still hopeful, seemed a bit more used to the idea that there was little chance of her mother surviving. The intensivist said they were going to take a tiny piece of her kidney and examine it under a microscope to try to find out if the cancer came from the lungs or whether the lungs and kidney are separate cancers. "We'll see what the test shows," said the intensivist, "if her kidneys get worse, we won't offer her dialysis, and if her heart stops, we won't treat it." "Will you ask us?" inquired the son-in-law. "It will be our decision," said the intensivist, "but we'll tell you." The intensivist explained that it might take a day or two for the test results to come back, and the husband said: "Let's see what the test shows and go on from there."

Later that day, I saw the younger daughter bringing in a little golden-haired boy to visit his grandmother; he looked about two or three. The patient's nurse, when asked her opinion, had said that, naturally, a mother knows her child best, but that she felt that seeing his grandmother in the ICU might not upset a child of that age, although an older child might have difficulties. The daughter seemed to be gradually becoming reconciled to the idea that her mother might not regain consciousness and that she would surely die, then, or in the very near future.

The following day, a renal consultant was at Mrs. Murray's bedside, conversing with the team making rounds. (He wore a dark suit, a formal shirt and tie, and highly polished shoes, which contrasted with the informally dressed intensivists, who generally wore short-sleeved sports shirts, cotton pants, and sandals.)[7] The consultant said that the respiratory support needed to help the patient breathe was too high for them to do a biopsy on the lung. The left kidney had a possible tumor, although it could have been an abscess. The patient had been given a sedative 48 hours earlier, and she was still deeply unconscious. She may well have had a stroke in addition to a pulmonary embolism. Later in the afternoon, I saw both daughters in the patient's room, lovingly combing her hair.

In the early evening, while typing my fieldnotes, I received a phone call: "We're having a meeting with the Murray family, would you like to come over?" I rushed to the hospital, a block from my apartment. Here is the description from my fieldnotes:

Off we went to one of the little conference rooms, the nurse, Sally, [the intensivist], me, the father, and two daughters. [The intensivist] went through the patient's history of cancer, and then told them that the CT had shown that material had gone not only to the patient's lungs but to her brain. He described what had happened, it went through a valve in the heart that is usually closed, but the pressure built up, so that these little clots went through. What this means is that not only will this cancer kill her, but if she recovers from this brain injury, and there's no guarantee that she will, she'll be seriously disabled. The daughter who had so much trouble grasping everything thought her mother had responded yesterday evening when she brought her child in; [the intensivist] told her it was probably a reflex. The daughter seems to have finally grasped that there's no hope for her mother. She's distraught, but no longer fighting fate. He told them that they would like to remove the breathing tube since that's all that is keeping her going right now, and she's not going to get any better. "So we're just keeping her alive for us, not her," she said, and [the intensivist] and her father and sister assented. The daughter wanted assurance that she wouldn't suffer and [the intensivist] gave it, telling her that they would give her morphine so that she would just go to sleep peacefully. [The intensivist] showed them the X rays and CT scans, and explained them very carefully, in English. He then told the family that they could think about this and meet with him whenever they wanted, later tonight or tomorrow morning. They decided that tomorrow morning at 11:00 would be a good time.

The next morning, which was a Saturday, the entire family was in the patient's room. The little waiting room was occupied so we all ended up in the large ICU conference room: the father, the two daughters, the intensivist on service that day, the nurse, and I. The intensivist repeated much of what yesterday's doctor had said: how Mrs. Murray had suffered a stroke on both sides of her brain, quite possibly when she passed out in the ward before coming to the ICU. I felt it must have been reassuring to the family to hear the same thing, in different words, from two different doctors; it was obvious that the doctors agreed on what happened. The intensivist talked about removing the ventilator tube and allowing her to breathe on her own. He said that she was less responsive today and, in answer to a question, said it might take a few hours after the ventilator was removed. The daughters and husband wept. But the younger daughter seemed reconciled to the idea of losing her mother. "She knows we love her and that we'll care for each other," she said. The patient's husband wanted to go back and say goodbye before the ventilator and lines were removed, which he did, kissing his wife tenderly. From my fieldnotes:

> The little daughter insisted on staying throughout the process of removing the vent and lines—which I suspect made it harder; the nurse and [intensivist] had to do everything *very* delicately as the daughter kept up a constant reassuring refrain, holding her mother's hand, stroking her shoulder, and kissing her: "It's all right mum, I'm right here. It's just a plaster (as they removed the tape holding the vent tube]. Good girl! I'm here, it's all right, I won't leave you." She sang a soft lullaby to her mother, as though she were her two-and-a-half year old son, as [the intensivist] and the nurse removed the vent and lines and prepared the bed so that the family could stand around the patient as she died. When we left the room, they were all around the bed.

The intensivist who conducted the family conference that Saturday reported that he had asked yesterday's attending what it was like having me sit in on the earlier conference with the Murray family. His colleague responded that he did not really notice me. He thought the family had not, either. Everyone was thinking about too much to notice an anthropologist sitting quietly in the corner.

"Do They Know It's a Total Disaster?"

On Tuesday night, Greg, the fellow who was on service, received five new admissions. Several were so gravely ill that there was a question of whether they would survive. The unit was so short of beds some patients were placed in the "Annex" around the corner from the rest of the West Ward.

On Wednesday morning, when I thought we had finished rounds in the West Ward, we went to the Annex. There was Miss Elspeth

Kline, aged 22, who had been kicked in the back of her head by a horse. A lock of blonde hair was evident under the bandages. The intensivists ordered various tests to assess the damage. "Dear me, what a disaster!" said that day's on-service attending. A conference with her family had been scheduled for that afternoon. "Do they know it's a total disaster?" asked the intensivist. "Not really," responded the nurse.

The family gave permission for me to sit in on the conference. Here are excerpts from my fieldnotes:

> The Kline family consisted of mother, wearing tasteful, expensive-looking gold jewelry, handsome father, pretty blonde teenaged daughter reading a glossy fashion magazine, son, and friend who were parking the car and came in late. The family looked tasteful, well-dressed, well-heeled. . . . [The intensivist] asked what they knew about their daughter's condition, and the mother gave a pretty good description of the fracture. She knew the injury but did not realize its severity. [The intensivist] told her that the daughter may die or be seriously disabled. They did a test that seemed to suggest poor electrical activity in the brain . . . which would mean severe disablement if she survived. The teenaged daughter, who had been paging through her glossy fashion magazine when [the intensivist] began to speak, was weeping with her sweater held up to her face; the mother wept throughout the conference, with her husband's hand on her shoulder. . . . It's not hopeless but it is serious, said [the intensivist]. They'll know more tomorrow. The mother had two final questions: Is she suffering? Will she suffer? The answer to both was No.

The following day, the patient looked slightly better. She was still unconscious, however, and the intensivists decided to give her 24 hours to see if she awakened. I dropped in to the room to say "hello" to her mother and sister. "This must be stressful for you," the mother said to me. (This thoughtful *politesse* seemed of a piece with the family's well-bred dress and demeanor.) I responded that I had a daughter and knew how I would feel in such a situation.

The test results, which arrived the next day, showed that the patient had severe brain injuries. The neurosurgeons, who had been consulted, felt it would be dangerous to operate on her. Her condition had obviously deteriorated. "She'll declare herself one way or the other," said the intensivist (which is medico-speak indicating that the patient's condition will either improve or go downhill toward death). I asked the nurse how Miss Kline got kicked—nurses always know such things—and she said it was a friend's horse. The patient worked at a stable weekends, and they were trying to get the horse in a box when it lashed out.

A family conference was scheduled for the following day, which was a Saturday. Earlier that afternoon, the on-service intensivist had held the final conference with the Murray family, where they had decided to let the patient go. He told me he had two additional end-of-life conferences to conduct before his meeting with the Kline family, and mentioned that still another patient had died at 8:00 A.M. that morning. Miss Kline then, was just one of a series of ICU "disasters."

The two teenaged Kline children were not present at this conference. The young man who had attended the previous conference was there, however; I surmised that he might be the patient's boyfriend. Here are excerpts from my fieldnotes:

> [The intensivist] was very direct. He went into the injuries, and how a large vein was almost entirely severed, and how the pressure on her brain stem had cut off many functions, and they could get no electrical activity, which meant the brain was not communicating with the body. The neurosurgeons had said that if they tried to operate, she'd die on the table. There's no hope, she's going to die, said [the intensivist] in a quiet, compassionate—but straightforward—way. The father wanted to know what would have happened if the brain stem had not been squeezed, and [the intensivist] said the injury was so great that it is possible it would have had the same outcome. The boyfriend wanted to know if the brain stem could regenerate, and [the intensivist] said no, it cannot. The mother put her arm around the shoulders of the boyfriend, and gave him a Kleenex from her purse. She seemed prepared for the outcome. Not resigned but prepared. There was some other hypothetical question, to which [the intensivist] responded, that the part of the brain that was injured, in addition to the squeezing of the brain stem, was the part that controlled speech and mentation. "I understand she was a bit of a high flier," he said, and the family members smiled. "She wouldn't be one anymore," he said.

The intensivist emphasized that the patient was going to die, in any case; it was just a question of timing. The mother said she had to talk to the two younger children, who had gone for a walk. They could not bear coming to the conference. "They know what is going on," she said, but she promised to talk to them before coming to a decision.

There was another conference with the family, later that Saturday afternoon that I did not attend. I was told that they insisted on continuing her treatment, so they kept her on the ventilator until she became brain dead the following day.

The intensivist who had conducted the final two Kline family conferences reported that he did stop her CSF drainage,[8] which may have hastened her brain death at 4:00 P.M. on Sunday. (If he had kept it going, there was a possibility the patient would have remained in a persistent vegetative state for some time.) "We had a bit of a ropy time at the end," he said. On Saturday night, the mother let them know that she thought they should have been given more time and more voice in decision making. The family questioned the patient's nurse and interpreted her response as showing lack of knowledge. Then when a nurse asked if they would like a chaplain, or minister, or priest, the mother felt this was insensitive, as though they were saying the patient's death was a sure thing. The mother made it clear that the family had high-ranking friends, that she had an influential job, and that the unit might hear more about this. "But I'm a big boy, I can stand it if I have to" said the intensivist. He said the unit had been backed up; they needed the beds and were turning down patients right and left. But he misread the family and had probably needed to take it slower. He had turned off the drainage without telling the family, which hastened her death. The family was not ready to consider her case as "hopeless," and focused on this. He was clearly trying to think about the situation: what he did wrong to so anger them, and how he might handle something like this another time. I myself sensed that the family almost had to be angry at someone; the death of a beloved, young "high-flying" daughter was so unbearable that someone had to be blamed.

Two months later, when the case was discussed at the meeting of the Bereavement Follow-up Team, Miss Kline's nurse indicated that the family had been critical and confrontational with her; she, too, felt that they needed someone to blame.

The intensivist who with a colleague made the final decision reported (in a subsequent e-mail):

> The place was a disaster that weekend. I did not have enough resources to manage the number of patients coming in (there were several other simultaneous disasters) and I (probably correctly) judged that the parents . . . would not have accepted removal of [the drain] or fully understood the irrelevance of it to the final outcome. This would have prolonged the patient's dying for at least another 3–4 days, and I frankly "needed the bed for other patients." I still feel bad about what happened and wish I had done it differently.

Here we see a conflict between scarce resources and the grief of a family unable to accept the loss of a beloved young daughter. We also see the pressure of *time:* Discussions of medical care often omit the crucial element of time, the fact that events press upon busy physicians, who must often make rapid decisions without the luxury of reflection.[9]

Would more time have helped? Would other patients, who needed these ICU beds to be given a chance to survive, have had to be turned away if this grieving family had been given more time to come to terms with the death of their daughter? In such a situation, there is no correct decision. Someone, a potential patient or Miss Kline's parents, will suffer, no matter what decision is made.

Weeks after Miss Kline's death, the intensivist gave me the outline of a medical presentation he had delivered some months earlier, where he argued that "early withdrawal of intensive therapy in severe brain trauma is not only justified but obligatory." Citing the medical literature, he stated that a test given Miss Kline (a SEP; Somatosensory Evoked Potential), which showed that electrical signals were not going from her brain to her body, had a 99.5 percent ability to predict long-term outcomes of patients with severe brain injuries.[10] "Poor outcomes" were defined as death, persistent vegetative state, or severe disability, involving loss of cognitive ability and emotional stability, reduced psychological well-being, unemployability, and social isolation. He gave statistics for 66 patients in the Auckland unit with severe brain damage whose treatment was withdrawn. Forty-four next of kin had been contacted six weeks later by the Bereavement Follow-up Team. Of these, 43 said they were well informed, and 41 understood the fatal sequence of events. He concluded that early withdrawal of treatment after a severe traumatic brain injury is justified ethically and legally, does not delay death, minimizes devastated survivors, minimizes waste of resources, and is understood and accepted by next of kin.

If indeed, Miss Kline was going to die from her terrible accident, or go into a persistent vegetative state, with the alternative being loss of ability to reason and relate emotionally, it is conceivable that she, herself, might have preferred not to survive. What her parents would have chosen, given some time to face her situation, cannot be estimated. Nor, can we know whether a few more days of reflection would have allowed them to come to terms with the loss of their cherished "high-flying" daughter.[11]

"He Wants to Live for His Child!"

As we made rounds one April morning, I learned that Mr. Sandur Rao, age 28, who had a drug-resistant organism, had been placed in a room away from the other patients. The patient had been at a private hospital before he choked on a potato chip and was sent to the Auckland ICU. He had originally suffered a heart attack, then a stroke; his legs were paralyzed and his arms so weak that he was unable to feed himself. He was diabetic and wheelchair-dependent. "Why was he accepted," I inquired. "I thought this was the kind of patient the unit didn't take." "That's because Giles was on," said the doctor leading rounds. I had been told that Giles was more likely to accept patients his colleagues might reject as unable to benefit from the services of the ICU, and slower to decide to move patients to comfort care. The intensivist said that the patient had a five-year-old child, and that it had been an arranged marriage. "Can you imagine saddling a woman with that!" she said.

A meeting with the family was scheduled for that afternoon. I will quote from my fieldnotes:

> I should think that for a young woman, it would be easier to have a dead husband than a paraplegic [paralyzed] chronic invalid. But of course I don't know Indian culture. Perhaps the death of her husband is the end of her life as a social being.
>
> The participants consisted of mother and father, who don't speak English; the sister, who did most of the talking; the wife, a small, dark-skinned shy-looking woman wearing no makeup (the sister is light-skinned and does wear makeup); the child, a girl of five who looked older; and an Indian nurse, who has been caring for him in the private hospital.
>
> According to the chart, this man has been incapacitated for eight years! What that means is that he well may have had this arranged marriage (he's 28) after he became an invalid.
>
> The nurse [his private nurse] said he had told her he was tired of living, that he suffered too much and wanted to die. "Oh, he only said that when he was joking," said the sister. The wife said she had never heard him say that. "He's so young, he's got to live," pleaded the sister. "If he were old, fifty or so, it would be different. Give him a few more days," she coaxed. "I just asked him if he wanted to get well to squeeze my hand, and he squeezed my hand." The [patient's] father spoke in an impassioned tone, which was translated into: "Give him the medicine that will allow him to live, that will make him better." The family didn't seem to hear a word [the intensivist] said about his condition or that the nurse said about his not wanting to live. "He wants to live for his child," said the sister, pointing to the child, "he loves it when he sees her."

The intensivist kept telling them that they were not sure that this almost quadriplegic (paralyzed in legs and partially in his arms) man had a quality of life that should be continued, and the family ignored his words. He finally agreed that they would keep him going another day and then discuss it again. The sister said her brother had to come to the meeting; he is the one who cares for the sick man and who knows about medicine. She tried to say that perhaps he could not come for two days, obviously to postpone any decision making. But the intensivist was obdurate and said that if the brother wanted to be part of the decision, he had to come the following day.

The intensivist who was on service the next day was sure that the family would disregard her because she is a woman. "All the Indian families are impossible!" she said, and a colleague indicated that the difficult cases tended to be Asian—Indian or Chinese. On morning rounds, the intensivist who was on service the previous day told the group that the family apparently went into the patient's room after the family meeting and asked him several times, "Do you want to live," and other questions of that sort, to be responded to by squeezing a family member's hand. When they left the room, the patient started hitting at the nurses. The doctor thought that the family's questions had led the patient to believe that they were trying to kill him. He told Mr. Rao that the nurses were his friends and commanded them, in the patient's hearing, to keep him alive.

When I mentioned this patient to a senior nurse, wondering how an almost quadriplegic man could have gotten his wife pregnant, she said that immigration will be at the bottom of it: The birth of a New Zealand child allows the entire extended family to stay in the country. "After all, someone else could have gotten the woman pregnant," she suggested. (We later learned that although he had serious medical difficulties eight years before, he did not become paralyzed until five years ago.) I mentioned noticing that the sister and patient are very light-skinned, which I understand is highly valued in Indian society, while the wife is dark-skinned; they may have been in a hurry to get a baby, and, when they arranged the marriage, went with whoever was available. "Now, they can set her on fire in the kitchen," said the nurse: "She's now expendable."

The woman intensivist had recruited a male colleague to attend the meeting with her the following day. This time, the sister's husband and the patient's brother—who looked as though he were in his late teens or early twenties—did the talking. The brother-in-law tried to use the breathing rate shown by the ventilator to demonstrate how well the patient was doing, but an intensivist told them that the machine set the rate, and the doctors could set it where they wished. The two doctors then emphasized that the problem,the patient aspirating a potato chip, indicated that he had weak lungs, otherwise he could have coughed the food out. But his breathing was weakened; this hospitalization would weaken his breathing further, and the doctors saw no possibility of his getting off the ventilator. (Treatment for this patient had been "limited," and the doctors had decided ahead of time not to give him a tracheotomy.)

The family kept saying, "But he wants to live, he said he wants to live for the child," pointing to the child as though this were an incontrovertible argument. They cycled round and round, apparently ignoring the intensivists' words, always bringing up the child, who they seemed to feel was their trump card. Gradually, however, it appeared that the family began to understand, very, very slowly.

I said, "She's a beautiful child," and the grandmother, who purportedly spoke no English, smiled proudly. "His will to live is so strong," said the brother. "We thought he was going to die, but he wanted to live, and look he did live, and even had a child." "His spirit may be strong but his body is weak," said one doctor. The sister kept asking for more time, and the doctors made it clear that more time would make no difference in his condition. They scheduled another meeting for the following day.

I could see how the family was gradually beginning to take in the information. The brother-in-law, who was obviously the senior decision-maker in the family, wanted to know what would happen if they removed the tube, and an intensivist responded that he would have trouble breathing and lapse into a coma and eventually die.

It was near the end of my stay in New Zealand, and I spent five days driving around the North Island (New Zealand is composed of three islands). Returning to the unit, I discovered that Mr. Rao was still alive. An intensivist said that they were learning more about him: He probably had severe preexisting illness and "was sitting on a knife edge; what happened to him had to happen one day." They planned to talk to his general practitioner to get an independent evaluation of how the *patient* felt about his life, as opposed to what the family said. Then an intensivist would talk to the family the following day.

I was getting ready to leave New Zealand, returning items various ICU staff members had loaned me, with an appointment to bring back the rented car. When I telephoned the intensivist, who planned to hold the third Rao family meeting, he reported that the patient had bitten a hole in his breathing tube. "He wants it out," said the doctor. He suggested I change the time for returning the car, so that I could attend the meeting, which I did. He then telephoned again. The patient had bitten another hole in his tube, and when the intensivist asked if he wanted it out, he assented.

A family meeting was scheduled for that evening; I had planned a good-bye dinner with the woman intensivist, so I did not attend. During dinner, the intensivist reported that she had talked to the patient's private nurse, who had been caring for Mr. Rao for some time, and learned that the family had not given the name of the patient's general practitioner, whom the doctors had wished to question about his condition and state of mind before coming to the ICU. Instead, they had given the name of *their* general practitioner. When questioned about his mental state, the nurse said he was often depressed and sometimes aggressive, and that intellectually, sometimes he seemed there and other times he seemed confused. She estimated that he had about 80 percent of normal intellectual function.

I kept calling the on-service intensivist from the restaurant, and learned that by 8:25 P.M. he had already held three meetings with the family and was about to go into the fourth. After the first meeting, they went to the bedside where the intensivist had asked the patient to squeeze his hand for "yes" and shake his head for "no." "Do you want the tube out?" the intensivist had asked. "Yes," responded the patient. "Do you want another tube put in?" "No." "If we take the tube out, you will probably die. Do you still want it out?" "Yes."

He held the second meeting with the disbelieving family, and then they all returned to the bedside, where they went through the same procedure with the brother-in-law holding the patient's hand. The intensivist asked the same questions and the brother-in-law received the same responses.

Then came the third meeting with the family. "Oh, he has a fever." "He's confused," with the women chorusing from the background: "He wants to live for his daughter." The intensivist, a wonderfully patient but persistent man, reported that he had told the family that if they felt he had a fever and was confused, they should not have questioned him. The family could not believe that the patient's responses were so different from those they had convinced themselves he felt. The intensivist said that the family was discussing what had happened, and that then they would hold their fourth meeting. He promised to call me the following morning to describe what happened.

The following morning, as I continued preparations for departure, a colleague, who had come to my apartment to pick up some borrowed household items reported that Mr. Rao was still on the patient list. "The fat lady has not yet sung," he declared.

After rounds, the intensivist on service the previous day telephoned, as promised, reporting that at the fourth meeting, the family had asked if he would keep the tube in until the next morning, and then ask the patient again if he wanted it out. The brother-in-law understood the situation, but the brother did not. The patient's breathing was poor, said the intensivist, and he was beginning to suffer. He told the family that if they left him until morning, he might be dead. They scheduled a fifth meeting for 10:45 P.M. and there, informed the intensivist that they wanted to remove the breathing tube. The intensivist said that he had been talking to them about the difference between what the patient wanted and what they wanted and how they had to honor the patient's wishes; this seems to have reached them. But they wanted time to go home, get some Coca Cola and Chicken McNuggets, which the patient loved, and give these to him. They scheduled another meeting, their sixth, for that evening, and when he asked, "Are you ready to remove the tube," they said, "No, not yet." At 12:45, the breathing tube was removed, and the patient was breathing on his own. He could not talk because his throat was swollen from the tube. The intensivist went home, but the family seemed quite happy at this stage. Somehow his brother had managed to communicate with him and this made him happy.

I left New Zealand the next afternoon. When the intensivist telephoned after morning rounds to report what had happened, he said that the patient was dying. When I remarked that the family seems to have used him as an endless resource, just turn the tap and there he is, the intensivist responded with great seriousness that this is not how he sees it: What *he* feels and what *the family* feels is less important than the welfare of the patient.

Another doctor telephoned an hour later with news of Mr. Rao. (The intensivists knew I was interested in the case, and kept me up-to-date.) The patient was alive, but he looked all pasty and was obviously dying. Since the ventilator tube had been removed, however, he was able to communicate with his family. The doctors kept him in the unit. They feel they can handle death better than any other service, and they knew the family and could help them deal with the death. I said that in the United States, the patient would probably have been in intensive care for eight weeks rather than eight days, and he would then have be given a tracheotomy and sent to an extended care facility, where he might have survived, paralyzed and on a ventilator, for some time. This might be what the family would have chosen—but would it have been the choice of Mr. Rao? In the United States, even among intensivists, moving a moribund patient out of the unit is, for many intensivists, a triumph. The quality of the dying and helping to alleviate the grief of the family are not perceived as part of the intensivist's job: This is the task of the chaplain or social worker.

9

Focusing on the Bottom Line

"No Margin, No Mission"

While conducting research, I spent a day each with five administrators at the Midwest medical center: the Chief Executive Officer,[1] the Chief Nurse Executive, the Chief Medical Officer, the Chief Operating Officer, and the chief of Surgery (the Surgeon in Charge). I told them that I wanted to learn more about the people whose decisions affected the day-to-day operation of the SICU; this would help me to understand the context in which the unit functioned. I spelled out the rules beforehand: I would meet each administrator when and where he or she wished; they could introduce me as they wished (as "Dr. Cassell," which was technically correct, or in any other way they felt was appropriate); they were free to ask me to leave whenever anything was discussed they they preferred I not hear; and I would stay with them until either I ran out of steam, they got tired of my company, or their day ended.[2]

Spending time with these administrators dispelled a host of prejudices and preconceptions. I had always assumed without reflection that the money that should have gone to hire additional nurses and raise their salaries, and similar projects, was being wasted by a host of overpaid VPs, pointy-headed little financial types who spent their time holding time-wasting meetings where they devised mendacious slogans, such as "we care," rather than supporting caring behavior throughout the hospital. I cannot say where

141

I got this impression. Perhaps nonverbally from the SICU doctors and nurses? I do not know.

I could not have been more wrong!

First of all, almost every administrator I met proved to be extraordinarily intelligent and dedicated—to the hospital and to his or her job. I had taken it for granted they would be a rather dim lot, astute primarily at political maneuvering. Not so.

I did find a radical disconnect between their concerns and those of the ICU personnel. There was one exception: the Chief Nurse Executive, who also held the title of Vice President of Patient Care. A former ICU nurse who had come up through the ranks, this woman was beloved by the nurses, who knew she was deeply attuned to the issues affecting patient care and the welfare of nurses.[3]

The Feds, the Regs, the Reimbursement Squeeze

The administrators were concerned with keeping the hospital afloat in perilous waters. The medical center was buffeted by forces from all directions.[4] From above came a host of federal regulations, costly to implement and often highly impractical, with little understanding of how hospitals function.

To give just one example: in 2003, new federal regulations to protect patient privacy required that every member of the staff who had "access to patient records," including secretaries and this anthropologist, were forced to take computer "training" in obeying federal regulations concerning "protected health information," and then pass a multichoice computer examination. The course was not uninformative, but the exam was rather simpleminded; a canny test-taker could figure out the system and pass without bothering with the course. No one seemed concerned whether the examinee passed or failed the test, the important thing was *to take the exam*, with dire legal penalties threatened for institutions whose employees did not comply.[5] The same unreflective literalness decreed that all patient records had to be kept in locked files; since many were presently stored in file cabinets with no provision for locks, new cabinets had to be obtained for sites throughout the hospital, at hundreds-and-thousands of dollars.[6] Moreover, discussing a patient outside that patient's room was now prohibited; this meant that an attending physician, rushing down the hallway to take care of some urgent concern, could not question a nurse or resident about a patient's condition without entering that person's room or knowing the room number: "What were the lab results of the tests for the woman in room number—?" Naturally, the person being questioned also had to remember the room number. Since HMO restrictions and government mandated-DRGs had increased the "throughput" of hospitalized patients, this would require strenuous feats of memory.[7]

At the same time, the administrators faced intense pressures for "accountability." Sociologist Carolyn Wiener documents what she calls "the elusive quest" for "accountability in hospitals."[8] She shows how tools, techniques, demands, and paradigms change, while the mirage of "accountability" hovers on the horizon, never quite reached by whatever techniques are presently mandated. Regulatory demands, she notes, are increasingly complicated and ever-changing. After five years of interviews and fieldwork in hospitals, Weiner is haunted by the nagging question: "Is all this effort geared toward making hospitals better or toward only making them *look* better?"[9]

Weiner discusses the work of the Joint Commission on Accreditation of Healthcare Organizations (JCAHO) indicating that, in 2002, the commission evaluated more than 17,000 health-care organizations in the United States, including more than 5,200 hospitals. She observes that in the early days of her research, its impact was described to her with "fear, awe, and, in some cases, loathing."[10]

I encountered "fear, awe, and, in some cases, loathing"—plus sheer terror—when the JCAHO inspectors' visits to the Midwest medical center were anticipated. An administrator hefted their manual of quality criteria: a loose-leaf folder, approximately three inches thick, which mandated everything from procedures to measurements (e.g., ICU storage shelves had to be a certain distance from the ceiling—an inspector might take a ruler to them, and if they were too close, the hospital might receive a demerit). I sat in on a meeting with a JCAHO inspector in the SICU. She was an intelligent perceptive woman who asked probing questions, but I was told that not every inspector is particularly intelligent or probing; some are small-minded and exceedingly literal. The JCAHO requirements may seem an odd mélange of thoughtfulness and Mickey-Mouse-pettiness to an outside anthropological observer, but this is a serious business. A hospital that fails its JCAHO inspection is threatened with losing its accreditation, which means that every regulation, however exacting and small-minded, must be adhered to scrupulously. This is not only a serious but also an extremely *expensive* business. An army of QA (quality assurance) "worker bees" (who, as Wiener notes, are likely to be seen as "killer bees" by some of the medical staff)[11] must labor year-round to assure that the JCAHO regulations are followed. Companies specialize in helping medical organizations fulfill the JCAHO and federal regulations; their highly paid consultants come in to train employees and set up mechanisms for compliance.[12]

In addition to the weight of "the regs," regarding quality and (so-called) ethics,[13] the hospital administrators faced severe constraints on reimbursement. Medicare and Medicaid regulations regarding reimbursement change constantly; changes generally involve increased paperwork (which necessitates more staff to handle it) and decreased reimbursement. These days, private patients are likely to have medical insurance, or belong to HMOs; their regulations also shift constantly, generally in the direction of decreased reimbursement. Medicare, Medicaid, insurance companies, and HMOs pressure hospitals to discharge patients as rapidly as possible—even if this policy means that patients will subsequently bounce back because they were released while still in need of skilled care.

The poorer the patients, the more likely they are to be uninsured, or covered only by Medicaid (which I was told reimburses approximately 20 cents on a billed dollar). The Midwest medical center was located in the center of a mid-sized city, close to pockets of urban poverty.[14] It was also relatively close to a lawless, and bankrupt municipality that sounded rather like Dodge City in an old-time Western: people always seemed to be getting shot, or bodies of people shot elsewhere were getting dumped there; many of these victims ended up in the Midwest ER, to be operated on by the trauma surgeons. Some adjacent hospitals had closed their trauma departments; others were considering doing so. I was told that 22 percent of the trauma patients had no insurance, and as a result, the trauma service had a yearly shortfall of $500,000 to a million dollars a year. Trauma had a 20 percent collection rate; the collection rate for the SICU was 40 percent, so it made money, but not a great deal. Consequently, the section handling trauma, burns, and (surgical) intensive care was the lowest-earning section in surgery.

Trauma patients tended to be disproportionately poor and African American. I was told that some doctors who sent their patients to the SICU lobbied for a separate waiting room for the families of trauma patients; they complained that the presence of these families was disturbing to the middle-class families of their patients.

Payments for trauma are handled differently in different regions. The Midwest medical center was located in a besieged city in an impoverished state; neither city nor state reimbursed the hospital for trauma care. A trauma surgeon reported that in San Francisco, the city pays the public hospital for trauma cases so the public hospital does not lose money, while in Louisiana the state pays the hospitals. In Texas, a case manager told me that although trauma loses money, it does not lose all that much; they find bits and pieces of funds in various places. She reported that their county has a tax fund that is used for care of indigent residents; one has to prove one is a resident to qualify, but it is not necessary to be an American citizen. Texas also has an Indigent Health Care network, and although poor counties such as theirs have less money, they get some funds from other counties, since patients are sent from remote localities to the only Level-1 civilian trauma center in south Texas.

The center-city location of the Midwest medical center generated a number of problems. Many comfortably situated families had moved to the surrounding suburbs, leaving the hospital with the poor, uninsured patients who lived relatively nearby. Hospitals with less urban locations competed with the medical center for insured patients. Not only were these hospitals easier for suburban patients and visiting families to reach, many had spacious campuses, with room to erect new buildings to meet growing demands, as medical technology expands and patients' expectations escalate. Although the Midwest center was constantly renovating and building, their expansion had severe constraints; new buildings had to be shoehorned into restricted spaces, and no grassy campus with room for new buildings existed. This meant that if, for example, the administrators wanted more private rooms to appeal to families who could afford to pay for them, they had to tear down existing structures, at a tremendous cost in money and disruption. The Midwest center had a lustrous reputation, but the old buildings possessed far too few private rooms, and the overcrowded garages contained too few parking spaces to comfortably contain the upscale cars and SUVs of middle- and-upper-class suburban patients and families.

The competition among the local hospitals for paying patients was ferocious. From the administrators' point of view, merchandising—using slogans such as "we care"—was one way of attracting such patients. The administrators spoke of the hospital's "mandate" to care for underserved patients. As one administrator said, however, during a meeting where the participants were weighing "scenarios" for the future, calculating how much margin the hospital needed in coming years in order to survive, "no margin, no mission!"

Let me note that the relationship between the Midwest medical school and the adjacent hospital has not been discussed because I know little about it. Hospital chiefs of service also held appointments in the medical school. The residency training programs were hospital based. I believe the medical school administered most, possibly all, the grant monies, but I am not entirely sure of this.[15] I was barred from one meeting, where the relationship between the hospital and the medical school was discussed; medical school administrators did not want me present. I did attend another meeting regarding transfer of hospital research facilities to the medical school, where ferocious bargaining was conducted about just who would pay for what. My impression is that the relationship between the two separate-but-conjoined entities was vexed, but I cannot say exactly why or how. It was clear, however, that the relationship did not ease the pressures on the hospital administrators and may have possibly contributed to them.

The disconnect between the concerns of the administrators regarding survival of the hospital and those of the doctors and nurses regarding patient care allowed for a great deal of maneuvering in the interstices between the two.

So far as I could tell, the chiefs of service were located in the space between administrators and practitioners. The chief had to answer to the administrators, showing that his department was a money-making concern.[16] He had to make sure that patient care was effective, contributing to the lustrous reputation of the medical center. He had to adjudicate between the different divisions and sections under him, receiving complaints, resolving clashes, doling out scarce resources such as office space and funds for secretarial help. To burnish the reputation of the medical center, the chief was expected to recruit, promote, and develop stars, who would garner international applause for their achievements and research. Each subspecialty should stand out. "Second best is not good enough!" declared the chief of surgery. One "report card" for each department was delivered annually through the ratings of *U.S. News and World Report;* these ranked not only hospitals, but also specific subspecialties within each hospital.

How much money each department brought in probably acted as another, internal, report card. Consequently, the chief might put pressure on his subordinates to spend more time on activities that produced revenue, and less time on those that did not. (Included in such pressure are salaries dependent on how much income each subordinate brings in.)

In this era of market measurements, "clinical productivity" is calculated in terms of income-generating activities. (Educational productivity cannot be measured, nor does it generate income.) Discussing such measures, disseminated by highly paid consultants who sell their business advice to medical organizations, Ludmerer observes:[17]

> A plastic surgeon generating large fees by performing routine cosmetic surgery on well-insured patients would be considered productive. A general surgeon or neurosurgeon at an urban teaching hospital performing lifesaving operations on young indigent trauma victims would not—even if that surgeon developed new approaches to the understanding and treatment of trauma and earned national acclaim as a leader in the field.

It is, perhaps, fortunate that *U.S. News and World Report* does not rate medical centers that lack a trauma center. This may well have protected the trauma surgeons from any temptation on the part of cost-cutting administrators to divest the hospital of this "unproductive" specialty.[18]

With productivity comes power. In the Midwest medical center, the money-losing trauma service was subsidized by other branches of surgery. I was told that the earnings of one man, with an international reputation in his surgical subspecialty, subsidized trauma. The general surgery division this man directed contained the burn/trauma/surgical intensive care section.[19] "He hates our section," I was told, and when I asked why, the response was, "because trauma loses money." This highly intelligent, charming, charismatic surgeon attracted private (and consequently paying) patients from a wide geographic area. He possessed enormous personal force and authority: A young attending trained at the Midwest center reported that although he now calls the other surgeons by their first names, he still addresses this man as "Dr. Croci." I suspect the young doctor's attitude combined respect and fear. Croci had the reputation of being subject to intense, terrifying rages. I never observed one, but a nurse described how he had "screamed" at her for five minutes.[20] She could not talk to him; it was obvious that he was unable to hear her: "His face was red, he looked as though he was going to stroke," she reported.[21] Dr. Croci possessed a keen political sense, and the rumor was that, when reprimanded by the authorities, he would threaten to take his patients and move to a competing hospital.[22] As a result, he was treated with care and permitted to get away with behavior that might be sanctioned in another less-charismatic, less-celebrated physician who was not so "productive."

A trauma surgeon told me that trauma was disrespected by the other surgeons. The trauma surgeons performed general surgery procedures on ER patients needing operations—especially evenings and weekends when the specialists did not want to come in. He had started turning these calls down. People were amazed. One Sunday a resident said to him: "You're Blue Service!" as though that meant he was at their disposal. And then at the M & Ms, the superspecialists would give them a hard time about the operations they *did* carry out; if he performed a colectomy, a colon surgeon might say, "That's not the way I would have done it." The other trauma surgeons wanted to do these general surgery cases; it helped keep them sharp. They told him he was supersensitive when he stayed up all night after "getting fried" at an M & M. "They take aim at us, we get it with both barrels," he reported. Trauma was the only section "in the red," and he was convinced that this affected everyone's attitude.

Focusing on Mission

There appeared to be less concentration on *margin* and more on *mission* at the Texas medical center. The hospital was in serious financial difficulties—I attended a meeting of administrators discussing this—but I saw no indication that the prestige of the trauma surgeons, or their patient-care decisions, were negatively influenced by the fact that so many of their patients were impoverished.[23]

In New Zealand, the intensivists were subjected to intense cost-cutting pressure by district health boards.[24] The politically appointed chairman of the Auckland Health Board asserted on national television: "Putting doctors in charge of hospitals is like asking rabbits to manage the lettuce patch."[25] So far as I could tell, however, this pressure had little effect upon the intensivists' powerful sense of mission.[26]

Does Margin Enable Mission?

Perhaps it is too temperate for me to describe "a radical disconnect" between the concerns of the Midwest administrators and those of the practitioners. It is conceivable that concentrating on margin does not *enable* mission, but instead, *nullifies* it. Surely a prestige system based primarily on money (even when concealed in a quasi-medical term such as "clinical productivity"), that allows money-makers a greater latitude for misbehavior, raises serious questions.

The head of the trauma section at the Midwest medical center disagrees with the notion that margin may nullify mission. In an exchange of e-mails comparing various hospitals and their constituencies, he wrote:

> At [Midwest] you had/have schizophrenia. This is no different than Hopkins [Johns Hopkins], the MGH [Massachusetts General Hospital], or any big famous teaching hospital. Some of the patients paid their bills, others did not. Keeping the bill-payers happy meant that the hospital could afford to care for the indigent. That's still true. People who admit lots of paying patients . . . still have substantial political power in the hospital. It's a pragmatic decision, not a moral one, to make sure that Orlando Croci's elective . . . case gets a bed while 25 people are in the ER waiting for an admission—Landy's patient is a well-insured patient who makes it possible for some of the other care to be delivered.
>
> Perhaps adopting business practices makes it seem more like a business. But without these practices, there is no margin and hence no mission. Like it or not, health care is very much a business and workers in the field are expected to be productive.
>
> A few minutes ago I went to [operate on] a . . . trauma [case]. Middle aged black man, multiple (like 14) gunshot wounds. No pulse or blood pressure, but a whisper of cardiac electrical activity. So they had a 13 minute transport time and brought him here. We had about 20 providers assembled downstairs in the ED [emergency department] and another 10 ready in the OR. Packs were opened, tubes arranged for use, etc. etc. He came in dead and stayed dead. But we spent considerable time and used substantial resources on someone who will not receive a bill, much less pay it. But the resource use is real, and has to be paid.

In contrast, Leon Eisenberg argues that the world of medicine and the world of business are incompatible.[27] The author, a psychiatrist at Harvard, observes that:

> Morale at teaching hospitals is lower than I can recall during my 50 years in academia. . . . Clinicians complain that . . . [they] can no longer offer their patients the time necessary to help them participate in their own care. They lament losing the opportunity to consult with colleagues about the complexities and challenges of the medical conundrums they are trying to solve. Because they are expected to generate clinical income, the time they devote to teaching is regarded as a debit item by the division chief.

He contrasts the ideal as discussed by Socrates: "No physician, *insofar as he is a physician*, considers his own good in what he practices, but the good of his patient" . . . [emphasis added by Eisenberg] with the pragmatics of the marketplace, as spelled out by economist Milton Friedman:

> Few trends could so thoroughly undermine the foundations of our free society as the acceptance by corporate officials of a social responsibility other than to *make as much money for their stockholders as possible.* [emphasis added by Eisenberg]

Eisenberg charges that pragmatism is replacing idealism in academic health centers, and that the language of covered lives, consumers, and providers is replacing his generation's use of the "quaint terminology" of patients and doctors. Words embody values, he observes, noting that "consumers had best beware of sellers; patients must be able to trust physicians."[28]

This "market medicine" approach is exemplified in a booklet that discusses the future of academic health centers (ACHs),[29] which asserts:

> To protect their societal mission, AHCs need to be more disciplined in applying sound business practices and more focused on the bottom line of their operations. Each *product line*, such as patient care, education, and research, must be as self-supporting as possible, and each program should be scaled according to its ability to sustain itself. [Emphasis mine.][30]

The Midwest administrators used a similar phrase, speaking of service lines, such as cardiac surgery, that should be "one of our biggest money-makers." Another service line, endocrinology, was estimated to have growth potential, since the current "epidemic" of obesity is likely to generate more cases of diabetes.

A surgeon friend of mine described with dismay how the chief of surgery at her renowned medical center had recently embraced the medicine-as-business model, reorganizing his department and forcing busy surgeons to attend retreats where "trainers" led the participants in New Age "sensitivity games." She commented: "Just when all those scandals and bankruptcies are making us question the corporate model, it's gaining a foothold in medicine."

Productivity can be broadly defined. It may include bringing in research grant money,[31] publishing in prestigious journals, and taking a leadership role in national and international medical organizations. Laudable as all of these activities are, they detract from the time and energy a physician has to spend on sensitive, compassionate, unhurried care of patients and communication with their families. Caring for and about patients and their families is relegated to nurses. Among physicians, caring becomes, as the title of a book asserts: a "lost art."[32] Rather than describing tangible, highly valued behavior by doctors, *caring* becomes a marketing slogan for hospitals.

An Ethic of Billable Hours

In 2001, a *New York Times* column on "Beliefs" cited an article by lawyer and theologian M. Kathleen Kaveny that discusses a worldview based on a "peculiarly lawyerly kind of time: 'billable hours.'"[33] One reason so many young lawyers are dissatisfied with their work, argues Kaveny, is that the regime of billable hours treats time as instrumentally rather than intrinsically valuable. What counts are the extrinsic goals of winning advantages for the client and profits for the firm; intrinsic satisfactions such as doing good work, nurturing younger associates, or contributing to the community cannot be translated into billable hours. The regime of billable hours levels time, flattening out its rhythms into a kind of "endless, colorless present." This ultimately erodes young lawyers' sense of self and isolates them from fellows. Resisting this worldview demands regular practices of reflection, ritual, and renewal—practices embodied in an alternative view of life's purposes that is shared and supported by a community of people, whether religious or secular.[34]

Medicine may once have offered such a community. The rigors of residency were the induction into that select group, which possessed its own rituals (such as "scrubbing," in surgery),[35] times of reflection (M & Ms where mistakes and deaths were discussed, with colleagues' comments on how to do better the next time),[36] and renewal (when new candidates were selected and meticulously trained). It was a community where compassion, caring, *and* technical expertise were valued. The celebrated physician Francis Peabody observed in 1927, "the secret of the care of the patient is caring for the patient." This is not to over-idealize the "old-time doctor," who possessed little technical knowledge compared to today's physicians. In addition, some doctors, medical schools, and proprietary hospitals were surely just as focused on money as are today's HMOs or giant health-care conglomerates.[37] Nevertheless, many doctors were convinced that medicine was a "calling" with a mission to care for patients. Many physicians still subscribe to this credo. Eisenberg cites a study that indicates: "In chronic disease, caring *about* the patient as well as caring *for* the patient can reduce pain and improve mobility while using the same medications that fail when patient and physician do not collaborate."[38] He quotes an article on "caring effects" that asserts:[39]

> Caring has been central to medical practice in all cultures throughout history . . . trade-offs between caring and technical expertise are not rational, necessary, or inevitable, provided that health services pursue human rather than commercial goals.

The anomie and dissatisfaction exhibited by residents reflect the ethic of billable hours. These values filter down from above. When the chairman of internal medicine at a prestigious medical school tells his faculty: "If you want to teach, do so at lunch—and keep your lunches short,"[40] medical students and residents get the idea: time is money. The same lesson is brought home when they observe attending physicians cutting corners as they make rounds and manage patient care, communicating with patients and families in a hurried fashion, if at all.[41] For many, medicine is no longer a noble "calling." Too many residents feel they are just putting in time, becoming trained in a specialty, to then work for HMOs, where, again, their billable hours will be carefully monitored with sanctions for those whose time is not sufficiently "productive." These young doctors have lost their sense of mission, a sense that is vividly portrayed in William Nolen's depiction of the rigors and rewards of his Bellevue surgical residency, or by the 80-year-old surgeon's response to his residency: "I *loved* it!" Money was never unimportant, but for many, it was not the primary incentive. In the early 1960s, a young internist, who felt that being a doctor was the most wonderful thing one could aspire to, remarked to me: "I love being in a profession where you can do well by doing good." (At the time, my father was helping to subsidize our family, and we had begun to repay his parents for the money they had borrowed for his medical school tuition.)

I have difficulty characterizing the ethic of billable hours as a moral economy. The profit motive, the responsibility (in Milton Friedman's words) "to make as much money for . . . stockholders as possible," is not *a* web of affect-saturated values—it is perhaps, in many ways, a *lack* of values. Capitalism may or may not stem, as Kaveny notes[42] from the Protestant ethic, as outlined in Weber's celebrated argument.[43] But in its present form, this view of time and of money is shorn of religious and value orientations. To paraphrase the words of the head of the trauma section, choices based on an ethic of billable hours are pragmatic not moral decisions.

Am I suggesting that the administrators I spent time with are corrupt or wrong-headed? No. So far as I can tell, they are honest and highly intelligent people trying to keep their medical center from succumbing to the forces that have closed so many institutions around the country.

Are they making the wrong decision by concentrating on margin, which inevitably restricts or corrupts mission? I do not know enough to judge. I cannot suggest an alternate course of action.

Eisenberg asserts:

> There is simply no way at all that an academic health center can maintain excellence in clinical care, serve impecunious patients, teach students and residents, advance the science of medicine *and* compete for price with hospitals that do not teach or do research and are willing to provide care no better than they need to, as long as they can do so at a profit.[44]

Discussing the "fragility" of academic health centers, Ludmerer emphasizes that their most important social functions—

> the education of future generations of medical professionals, the discovery of new medical knowledge, the provision of highly specialized services (such as the care of patients with severe burns, complex trauma, and AIDS), and the care of poor and uninsured persons—[are] not income-generating activities.

The disquieting possibility exists that, in attempting to compete with for-profit hospitals, academic health centers will become more like them. As the *means* change, with an increasing focus on the bottom line, the *ends* may become corrupted.

Perhaps it is the system that is flawed—even corrupt. Government regulations, designed to care for the "underserved," are formulated, ringed round with so many caveats, complications, and cost-cutting mechanisms that it becomes a Sisyphean task to serve the underserved. Mechanisms to catch cheats, and implement ethical imperatives are so Byzantine and, at the same time, literal that the only people who can negotiate them with ease are dishonest physicians and health organizations. Cheats have no trouble with "regs"—they just lie.

The American health-care system is fragmented and disordered. Regulations and funding mechanisms differ from state to state. It has been estimated that in any given year, one-third of the U.S. population below the age of 65 is inadequately insured.[45] The United States is the only industrialized nation that tolerates this dismal state of affairs in which millions of children are at risk. Medical economist Ewe Reinhardt charges:

> As a matter of conscious national policy, the United States always has and still does openly countenance the practice of rationing health care for millions of American children by their parents' ability to procure health insurance for the family or, if the family is uninsured, by their parents' willingness and ability to pay for health care out of their own pocket or, if the family is unable to pay, by the parents' willingness and ability to procure charity care in their role as health care beggars.[46]

This is the environment in which the Midwest medical center struggles to survive, in which the intensivists struggle to give technically brilliant and clinically informed care, in which families see their loved ones hooked to machines, cared for by overburdened physicians and residents who too frequently lack the time and training to communicate with them directly and openly, and to help them make the terrible decision (that I, for one, believe no family member should be forced to make) to "pull the plug on your brother."

10

The Dominion of Death

And death shall have no dominion.
Dead men naked they shall be one
With the man in the wind and the west moon;
When their bones are picked clean and the clean bones gone,
They shall have stars at elbow and foot;
Though they go mad they shall be sane,
Though they sink through the sea they shall rise again
Though lovers be lost love shall not;
And death shall have no dominion.

—Dylan Thomas[1]

In medical science, the unlimited battle against death has found nature unwilling to roll over and play dead. The successes of medicine so far are partial at best and the victory incomplete, to say the least. The welcome triumphs against disease have been purchased at the price of the medicalized dehumanization of the end of life.

—Kass, 2002[2]

An American SICU is a miraculous place to be if you are a patient with reasonable odds of surviving. All the resources of technology, medical knowledge, and drugs, will be brought to bear to help you walk out of that door back into your life. If you are likely to die, however, an American ICU is a terrible place to depart, surrounded by machines, with tubes in every orifice, unable—because of sedation

155

and the ventilator tube in your throat—to communicate with those you love and say good-bye.

"Cheechee"

American doctors tend to be uncomfortable with dying patients. A British physician observes:

> In the UK we strive less officiously to keep alive. This is not callousness but stems from a different attitude to death. American physicians seem to regard death as the ultimate failure of their skill. British doctors frequently regard death as physiological, sometimes even devoutly to be wished.[3]

This attitude is slowly changing, but it is still a rare American physician who sees his or her role as helping a terminal patient to die well. Since data suggest that 20 percent of all American patients who die do so in the ICU, this is a serious concern.[4] Too often in ICUs, "heroic" doctors persuade patients or their families to continue treatment that many skilled observers find cruel, useless, and unnecessary. Some residents employ the term "flogging" to describe use of technology to prolong dying. The French have an even more graphic phrase: *acharnement thérapeutique. Acharnement* is what an animal does to its prey before devouring it.[5] In an ICU studied by Zussman, the residents described such technological abuse of the body as "cheechee," referring to an old, and not particularly amusing joke, which he cites in one of its briefer versions:

> Missionaries in a tribal land are captured by the natives and brought before the chief, who gives them a choice of "cheechee or death." The first missionary chooses cheechee. He is then set upon by the group, tied to a pole, and beaten by each member of the tribe. The rope is then tied around his hands and he is dragged about a mile, losing bits and pieces of himself. Finally, he is thrown over a ravine. The second missionary, asked what he chooses, says, "I never thought I'd say this, but I would prefer death." The chief says, "Yes, but first a little cheechee."

Zussman comments:

> The joke is a precise metaphor. Death is certain. What appears to be a choice is really no choice at all. But death cannot come quickly. In the joke it must be preceded by "cheechee." In the ICU, it must be preceded by treatment.[6]

Here is one such case. (Let me note that that although the ICU attendings, residents, and nurses perceived this as flogging or cheechee, the patient's surgeon construed this treatment quite differently.)

During my first month in the Midwest ICU, a young attending physician, who knew I was interested in end-of-life issues, called my attention to a patient: Mr. Dalby was a 46-year-old man who had received a second liver transplant two days earlier. He had an infection and acute liver rejection, and was on what was described as a "rapidly spiraling downhill course." Said the attending: "Basically, he's dying." His only possibility of survival was a third transplant, and the attending indicated, "that's really not an option." A resident, presenting Mr. Dalby's case during morning rounds, reported that only the patient's young heart and lungs were keeping him alive. The attending said that he had held a long conversation with the family during which, being "very optimistic," he estimated that Mr. Dalby had a 5 percent chance of surviving. The family wanted the patient made comfortable, and that was the ICU doctor's goal: to make him comfortable.

A few days later, Mr. Dalby's condition had improved and the surgeons discussed the possibility of performing a third liver transplant. After another relatively stable day and night, the ICU attending increased the patient's probability of receiving a third transplant from 5 percent to 15 percent or 20 percent. The surgeon declared that he would give Mr. Dalby one more day, and if he looked good, his team would consider a third transplant.

Passing the patient's room that afternoon, I encountered a nurse with her arm around the shoulder of his wife. She was listening as Mrs. Dalby told her that *she* never could stand having such terrible things done to her. "But what did he want?" asked the nurse in an understanding, comforting tone. She listened and reassured and, before leaving, brought in a box of Kleenex for Mrs. Dalby.

This occurred on a Friday. The following Tuesday, I learned that Mr. Dalby had developed VRE (Vancomycin resistant enterococcus), a deadly bacterium. An intern described it as "the most evil bacteria there is, circulating in his blood." Despite this setback, the transplant surgeons had the patient listed for a third transplant. The nurses reported that they had never had a patient in the ICU who had survived VRE; they felt the entire situation was abominable. "It's 100 percent fatal," said one nurse. The original plan was that if Mr. Dalby grew VRE out of his blood, the doctors would stop treatment. Despite this, the surgeons decided to go ahead. He was "on the list" (of patients scheduled to have liver transplants when and if a suitable organ became available), and if someone expired very soon, he would get a liver; the criterion is that the sickest patient gets the transplant, and

Mr. Dalby was the sickest. "Let's hope no one has an auto accident for a while!" commented one disapproving nurse.

Later, some nurses and I talked with the chaplain, who had just spent an hour with the Dalby family. The patient was unresponsive despite having received no sedatives for some time. He had started having seizures and the doctors worried that his sepsis (infection) might have affected his brain. The patient's wife was ready to "let him go," reported the chaplain, but the transplant surgeon kept encouraging her, saying that he had patients like her husband who are walking around today. The wife did not want to make the wrong decision. The transplant team is notorious for this kind of behavior, reported one nurse; when a wife wants to let her partner go, they say "How dare you!" The chaplain kept asking if anyone knew the odds and could cite them to the family. "If it's 50–50, it might be worth going for it, but if it's less, perhaps not," he said. It was apparently far less than 50–50. No one wanted to give exact odds, although one nurse guessed that the patient had about a 1 percent chance of surviving.

The chaplain observed that the family knew the transplant surgeons; they were the ones who talked to family members and put tremendous moral and emotional pressure on them: "How can you let him die!" In contrast, the patient's wife and brother wondered: "How can we waste a liver? He will be given a liver that, otherwise, might save another person's life." "Letting someone go is such a terrible decision," said the chaplain, and if a surgeon is putting pressure on the family to keep on trying, it is hard to go against him. The chaplain was very upset. He described the family as "going through a tunnel of hurt."

That evening the doctors took an EEG, tracing the electrical activity of the brain; this showed seizure activity. The doctors concluded that the patient had "end-stage sepsis," which had affected his brain, and would not recover. After discussing the matter with the family, the doctors and family agreed to put the patient on "full comfort measures" (this meant giving him everything necessary to keep him comfortable, but not coding if his heart stopped). The patient was taken off the ventilator and died soon afterward. I learned that the transplant surgeon, discovering that the patient had been given morphine and taken off the ventilator, had exclaimed: "I consider that euthanasia!"

After observing the case of Mr. Dalby and other patients in similar situations, it occurred to me that it might be a good idea to spend time observing some transplant surgeons. It was obvious that the world looked very different from their eyes.

"Every Single Person We Care for Would be Dead Without Us!"

An ICU attending physician described the first man I spent time with as "the ideal surgeon." He has "wonderful hands, marvelous clinical ability, and enormous knowledge," said the attending. "The only thing is, he doesn't look the role." He was right in all respects; this rather small, boyish-looking man was a fantastic surgeon and a warm, thoughtful human being.

I liked all three transplant surgeons I spent time with and had a wonderful time observing them at work. Transplant surgery is *exciting!* What an incredibly high-adrenaline pursuit.

I learned that transplant surgeons went, themselves, to retrieve the organs they used, and I told the first man that I would like to accompany him when he obtained organs. (The term doctors use to describe this is rather grisly: Surgeons *harvest* organs.) One Saturday afternoon, I received a phone call. I will quote from my fieldnotes:

At about 12:15, after making chicken stock, baking bread, shaping crab cakes, and having lunch . . . the phone rang. "Joan, this is Jim Sanderson [the surgeon] . . . we're going to get a liver, do you want to come?" We were met by several others [a chief resident, an intern, and members of the heart transplant team]. . . . We were leaving from [a small local] airport. Sanderson said they were having an air show . . . and all those expensive Air Force jets would be diverted while we take off. The priorities for planes, he said, were Air Force 1, Air Force 2, and then chartered transplant planes.

Riding an ambulance, with the siren going, is definitely the way to go. Cars get out of the way. When they don't, the siren can be exchanged for a sort of tweety sound, and also a commanding deep honk. We got there *fast.* Sanderson said that's the most dangerous part of the trip, the ambulance ride.

In the ambulance, Tod [the chief resident] and Sanderson talked about fellowship training (Tod is applying for a cardiothoracic fellowship). . . . Tod is working 7 days a week right now. Apropos of Tod's schedule and the fellowship training, Sanderson said to me: "That's what I mean about paying your dues" [he had mentioned "paying dues" earlier in the week].

There were two little planes waiting for us. . . . Most of us got into one plane, which was a "Satellite 65," a Sabreliner jet built to military specifications. . . . The others took a prop jet, which takes 7 minutes longer to get to [our destination]. Lots of bags and insulated cases came with us.

We were getting a liver and a kidney, possibly two kidneys. "Steve's going to put the liver in" said Sanderson [Steve Harmon was the chief of liver and kidney transplant]; "I'll put in the kidneys."

Sanderson said that the plane costs about $17,000 an hour, the ambulance rental is expensive, they have to pay the hospital for using their OR. He estimated that it costs about $40,000 to harvest a liver. All in all, it's about $150,000 [to perform a liver transplant]. Insurance pays. Medicare pays just about enough to cover the costs of the procedure. Medicaid pays 19 cents on the dollar. Interestingly, the cadaver-donor was referred to throughout as the "patient."

Sanderson and Tod talked about flying at night, through storms, to retrieve livers. It can be dangerous, said Sanderson, who is clearly trying to indoctrinate me into their mystique. . . . He spoke of "risking our lives." "Now you can see why we're so invested," he said.

We took another ambulance to the hospital, arriving . . . at about 2:20. It's a small private hospital.

The first thing we do said Sanderson is to check the death certificate and the consent form; he then checked the ID bracelet to make doubly sure he had the right person.

It seemed to me that they opened the patient and got down to the organs more rapidly than usual. I guess they didn't have to worry about doing it so that she could be put back together again?.

The table was surrounded by surgeons. The heart team removed, inspected, and rejected the patient's heart as unsuitable for transplantation and left the room. Sanderson and Tod kept on working.

The liver looked as though it was almost out. . . .. They packed the cavity with ice as they worked. They were now disconnecting the veins, artery, and bile duct. At 4:25 it was out and Sanderson called for the "liver bucket." The liver was placed in a basin on a table, and Sanderson rinsed it and examined it, running some sort of fluid into the veins and artery and then drying them off.

Sanderson returned to the operating table. (The liver was now in a plastic bag in the basin.) Suddenly, after watching all of this, I realized: this woman is *dead*. I don't remember ever seeing a dead person before.

The surgeons were working away. . . . Was it one kidney or two, I wondered. It was 4:42. Obviously one, since Tod was still working, while Sanderson scrutinized the kidney at the table against the wall. It was in an envelope of fat. He measured it with a little ruler, and a woman from the team, took down all the information. He then took the other kidney, which had been removed, and measured it. Tod was still working at the operating table. When I asked, Sanderson said he was removing the ileac artery and vein; they use these for grafts in emergencies.

Finally, we were finished. We changed and went to the ambulance. . . . We loaded everything on the plane and took off.

Tod was on the phone arranging for people to assist at the various procedures. . . . Sanderson was doing both kidneys, one after the other. The second was going to a child, a girl who has been on dialysis for 6 years. Being on dialysis is a full-time career, said Sanderson. For mother as well as child, I said, and he said the mother seems to be out of the picture, it's the grandmother who's caring for the kid.

We got back to the medical center by another ambulance. We arrived at about 7:15. Sanderson and the chief resident would spend probably much of the night operating. I hotfooted it back to my car and home. Yeah, they pay their dues, and they're high.

I learned that Dr. Sanderson was up until 3:00 A.M. transplanting the two kidneys. The following Tuesday, I met the African American 11-year-old who had received one. She seemed extremely knowledgeable about medical procedures, asking probing questions, which Sanderson responded to with warmth and understanding. Sanderson introduced me as "Dr. Joan" and told her I had been there when he obtained the kidney. During his rounds, he chatted with a nurse, who seemed to be part of the transplant team, who exclaimed: "Isn't it exciting about Clifford! He's been on the list six years." "He's a good guy," responded Sanderson. I reflected: If they know their patients six years before they get transplants, they surely do *know* them.

The trip to obtain the organs reminded me of a classic movie I had seen years before at a film festival, about bringing the serum for a sick child from or, perhaps to, Nome, Alaska; it involved snowstorms, dogsleds, and a tiny plane battling the elements to save the child's life. When I mentioned carrying the serum to Nome to the chief of transplant, he said, "Yes, it's a bit like Sir Lancelot going to get the Grail, and returning with it."

I attended two meetings of the liver transplant team, which included a psychiatrist, a renologist (specializing in liver disease), a financial expert, transplant nurses, and the surgeons. Here, they discussed who was going to be put on "the list" for a transplant and what listing they were given. (Medical insurance was one of the factors considered; benefits had to cover the cost of possible complications as well as costly immunosuppressive drugs that had to be taken for the remainder of a patient's life.) A score of 1 means that person is likely to die soon without a transplant; these people are given pagers, which go off if a compatible liver becomes available. Some patients, however, may be on the list for years before a liver becomes available. Powerful stuff. These doctors do, in a sense, "play God."

I also observed three transplants: a liver transplant and two kidney procedures. The liver transplant (from a living donor, a section of whose liver was removed in the adjoining operating room) was scheduled for 7:30 A.M.. The patient was on the table being "prepped" at 8:35, and I left the OR at 3:30 P.M., when they assured me that they were closing. I was so exhausted I could hardly stand; adrenaline and years of training must have kept the surgeons going.

Chatting with me before the procedure began, the surgeon remarked that they had a special relationship with their patients. "Every single person we care for would be dead without us," he declared. Transplant surgery is at the cutting edge, he said, and the procedures keep getting harder. (I surmised that the difficulties probably multiplied as they attempted increasingly daring procedures on a wider range of patients.)

The patient, Mr. Bordo, aged 49, suffered from end-stage liver disease, alcoholic cirrhoses, and hepatitis C, which I was told is incurable and extremely transmittable. "Is it like operating on someone with AIDS?" I inquired, and the surgeon said it is worse than AIDS because there are no drugs for it. "It gives you a different perspective on things when you know you're operating on someone who can kill you," he said.

The operation was long—some time was spent waiting for the section of liver to be removed from the donor (the patient's cousin) in the next room—but the patient made an uneventful recovery, spending a day in the ICU before being sent to the floor. The ICU physicians and transplant surgeons agreed that most transplant patients do have a smooth postoperative course, leaving the unit the day after the procedure.

Four months later, however, Mr. Bordo was back in the ICU with esophagitis, gastric and duodenal erosions, and peritonitis. "Whatever's going on with this guy, it's not [getting] better," said the ICU attending. After a month in the unit, Mr. Bordo was still very sick. Mrs. Bordo requested a conference with the transplant surgeon; the patient's sepsis (infection) was worsening, he did not respond to stimuli, and his wife could not bear seeing him that way. She wanted to ask the surgeon to shift to "comfort measures only." When the surgeon arrived, he talked to the wife outside the patient's room.[7] According to a nurse, who was present throughout their conversation, he told Mrs. Bordo not to listen to the ICU doctors, that he knew the patient's liver and knew he would recover. (The transplant surgeon had passed certifying boards in critical care and told me that he knew more about intensive care for transplant patients than did the ICU attendings. He may well have, although he probably lacked the time to keep up with the literature, as did the ICU doctors.) "I think we can fix this thing by taking him back to the OR for a washout," said the surgeon. Mrs. Bordo responded that all she wanted was for her husband to be comfortable. She inquired: "How long can someone survive on a "vent" [ventilator] like this?" The surgeon responded: "Oh, I don't know—we don't just turn off the vent because people are bored." The nurse reported that the patient's wife and daughter were so tormented that she had to take them into the small conference room generally used for family meetings, for some "quiet time." Speaking of the surgeon, the wife said: "How can he do this to me? I feel pulled in 10 different directions!"

Mr. Bordo was brought back to the OR, an abscess was found and drained, and his condition improved slightly. His mental status was poor, however. "I just wish he wasn't as squirrely," said the attending on service that week, who predicted that despite the surgeon's optimism, the patient would not leave the hospital; if this were his patient, he said, he would let him go.

The following month, the patient was still in the ICU. His indicators of hepatitis C had tripled from those taken the previous year. Mr. Bordo was dying from progressive hepatitis C disease, said that week's on-service ICU attending. The ICU team discussed various therapies. "What we're doing now is like rearranging the deck chairs as the Titanic sinks," remarked the attending. A resident, who prided herself on "telling it like it is," said she had informed the family, "We've done everything, tried everything, and made no difference in his condition." His hepatitis C measures were soaring, the team despaired of "weaning" him from the ventilator, and the ICU doctors considered telling the family he should be sent to a chronic care facility.[8]

After 65 days in the ICU, Mr. Bordo was accepted by a unit in the hospital that cares for patients who are still dependent on the ventilator. Two weeks later, when I inquired, I was told that the patient had been discharged from this unit, and was walking![9]

The transplant doctors, then, were justified in holding on. Transplant surgeons are in the business of providing miracles, of giving life when there is almost no hope. To do this, they have to be more confident than most surgeons, to feel that *they* hold the key to life and that *they* will walk the patient through the valley of the shadow of death. They cannot bear anyone, including family members, questioning them and their judgment. It is this confidence that gets the patient through—when he or she gets through.

That, of course, is a crucial question. How much "cheechee" must how many patients like Mr. Dalby endure so that a Mr. Bordo can survive? (Not only the patient endures cheechee, the family suffers as well.) Perhaps it is not perceived as cheechee when the patient recovers; it then can be defined as prolonged and occasionally painful therapy.[10]

Who should make these terrible decisions? And what criteria should be used to decide?

"The Temptation to Slash and Suture Our Way to Eternal Life"

Transplant surgeons possess the surgical temperament par excellence.[11] Describing the "American frontier value system" prevalent among transplantation and artificial organ pioneers, sociologist Renée Fox and biologist Judith Swazey describe these men (and most are men) as: "heroic, pioneering, adventurous, optimistic, and determined." They note, however, that there is a dark side to their ethos, which "often involves a bellicose, 'death is the enemy' perspective; a rescue-oriented and often zealous determination to maintain life at any cost; and a relentless, hubris-ridden refusal to accept limits." Leaving the field, after 40 years of research for Fox and 24 for Swazey, they state:

> By our leave-taking we are intentionally separating ourselves from what we believe has become an overly zealous medical and societal commitment to the endless perpetuation of life and to repairing and rebuilding people through organ replacement—and from the human suffering and the social, cultural, and spiritual harm we believe such unexamined excess can, and already has, brought in its wake.

They quote theologian and ethicist Paul Ramsey, who warns in biblical terms against "the triumphalist temptation to slash and suture our way to eternal life."[12]

The conflict between the search for medical progress and the human suffering this search can generate is discussed in a *New Yorker* magazine profile of Francis Moore, one of the most renowned surgeons of his time (who died in the 1970s). As chief of surgery at Harvard, Moore led his department in perilous experiments that pioneered innovations including organ transplantation, heart-valve surgery, and the use of hormonal therapy against breast cancer.[13] Until late in life, Moore exemplified the "dangerous dauntlessness" that Fox and Swazey question.[14] "Death, he argued, must never be seen as acceptable. Confronted with a dying patient, he did not hesitate to consider the most outrageous proposals."[15] Later in life, however, Moore had second thoughts about the ethics of what he, and others like him, were doing and began to wonder whether science was not keeping people alive too long. The author of the profile, Atul Gawande, himself a young Harvard surgeon, wonders which Moore was the better, the dangerously dauntless one, or the later Moore who had ethical qualms about such experimentation. He confides: "Strangely, I find that it is the young Moore I miss—the one who would do anything to save those who were thought beyond saving."

The author's preference is not at all strange. He is a *surgeon*. Gawande was admitted to the prestigious Harvard training program because he displayed "the right stuff."[16] A system of rewards and punishments nurtured his activist, aggressive, heroic stance.[17] Surgeons do not just stand there and contemplate ethical distinctions, they *do something*. When I presented my research findings to a group of surgical residents, a significant minority objected in their critical evaluations of the lecture to the fact that *I gave them no suggestions about what to do*.

Could surgeons change? Should they change? Should they become less aggressive, better able to communicate with patients and families, more interested in and knowledgeable about caring for dying patients? Or are they superbly selected and trained to do what they do: battle death with all the technological armamentarium modern medicine has to offer?

American surgeons are, perhaps, more—well, *surgical*, than surgeons in other countries. "The imperative to intervene," says Payer, was and is still critical to American physicians' professional identities.[18] If "American physicians seem to regard death as the ultimate failure of their skill," surgeons are the most American of physicians.[19] As the attitude of the younger Francis Moore's was described: *death is never acceptable*.

Tragically, we all know that attempting to slash and suture our way to eternal life leads to damnation and suffering, not to the defeat of death. Death comes, but first a little cheechee.

Some surgeons have taken steps to change the culture of American surgery. Geoffrey Dunn, a third-generation surgeon who edits a section in the *Journal of the American College of Surgeons* on "Palliative Care by the Surgeon," argues that surgeons must change to meet the changing demands and expectations by patients, and that the traditional heroic authoritarian surgical model fits poorly in today's more egalitarian ethos.[20] A Surgical Palliative Care Workgroup has been established to facilitate change and devise guidelines for surgeons on how to communicate with families and care for dying patients.

Today, however, surgeons interested in delivering compassionate, informed care to dying patients and their families are in a distinct minority. Surgical M & M conferences still focus on blaming and shaming colleagues who did not conduct the battle against death to the bitter end. Death is unacceptable. Cheechee is unmentioned.

Discussing these struggles about limiting or withdrawing aggressive treatment would seem to portray ICU physicians as compassionate healers who would never think of flogging a dying patient. Sadly, this is not so.

The RUB, the Risk of Unacceptable Badness, was considered by some but not all intensivists in the Midwest SICU. It was never discussed as such, but as the patient's potential quality of life after leaving the unit. The notion seemed far more established among the critical care doctors I encountered in New Zealand. Variation in how dying patients are treated exists not only among the intensivists in the Midwest ICU, but throughout the United States and the Western world.[21]

In April 2003, the International Consensus Conference on Challenges in End of Life Care was convened in Brussels, Belgium, to discuss the problems posed by the fact that today, more and sicker patients survive longer in ICUs, often kept alive primarily by sophisticated technological systems. After listening to two days of presentations by experts, a 10-person jury was charged with answering a series of questions about ICU care at the end of life. Their response to the first question: "Is there a problem with end-of-life care in the ICU?" was "Definitely yes!" The jury noted the tremendous variability in the practices of end-of-life care, both within and between countries, in the frequency with which decisions are made to forgo life-sustaining treatments, the timing of withdrawal of treatment, the types of treatments withdrawn, and the manner of withdrawal.[22]

Lord Kelvin's Fallacy Revisited

One challenge in making decisions at the end of life is posed by the difficulty of establishing beforehand just who is likely to die and who has a good chance to survive in a condition they, themselves, might find acceptable. Just what is a "good" chance? The statistical odds of survival refer to a group of patients suffering from a certain condition. Deciding how one particular patient will do is often almost impossible.[23] When does one cross the fine line dividing resolute efforts to keep a patient alive, deploying all the resources available to modern medicine, from cheechee, the use of technology to prolong a patient's dying?

This is an issue that has been much discussed among doctors, often in terms of *medical futility:* When is continued aggressive care futile? Various definitions of "futility" have been advanced and contested, as has the utility of the concept.[24] A New Zealand intensivist objects to the term "medical futility" for a number of reasons, including "faint resonances of abandonment" and the fact that futility is discussed in terms of the doctors' privilege to define it, ignoring interactions with the family.[25] He prefers the concept of a reasonable decision or, better still, a decision that it is *unreasonable* to continue aggressive care. A similar suggestion was offered by a British intensivist during the Brussels' end-of-life jury deliberations. As the New Zealand doctor pointed out, however, the concept of "a reasonable person" is enshrined in British common law, with echoes and meanings that may escape those who live under different legal systems. For example, the American legal system is based in part on the notion of damages: Did the doctor damage the patient by treating against that patient's will or withholding treatment? Consequently, what a "reasonable person would decide" does not necessarily have the same significance for American and European physicians. A reasonable surgeon? A reasonable intensivist? A reasonable family—from which ethnic background: Chinese, Indian, African American, Spanish Catholic, white Anglo-Saxon Protestant?

American deliberations focus on *certainty*, taking place in a legalistic and rule-bound context, says the New Zealand intensivist, who declares: "'This paralyzing discomfort with inherent uncertainty' is quintessentially American." He continues:

> To be crudely blunt, we [in New Zealand] accept that by making decisions prior to decomposition of the body, there will always be times when the patient "might have survived" if intensive therapies continued "forever." Does that make such a decision "wrong"? I think not. . . . By making the decisions take place in a transparent way (obvious to the nurses, the families and other involved staff from outside the [ICU]), we think that we "continuously test the waters' of 'societal reasonableness' (which does, of course change over time). . . . We focus more on "it is unreasonable to continue" than "we should continue because there is a reasonable chance" . . . if you use a term like "reasonable chance" then someone (especially in the US) will want to know what percentage that term corresponds to.

He notes that their approach in New Zealand, thinking in terms of unreasonable to continue, represents a "personal moral discomfort with continuing" as opposed to a reasonable chance, which can stand for "a certain level of statistical certainty."[26]

The intensivist notes, as I did when conducting this research, that cultural differences affect doctors' practices *and* patients' expectations. He comments: "How can there be a societal agreement on 'reason-ableness' when [American] society cannot even agree to provide some level of 'universal healthcare entitlement' to all its citizens?" He con-cludes, as did I, that not only administrative models (open, closed, semi-closed ICUs) and doctors' values affect medical decision making, but also what he calls "societal myths" and what I characterize as moral economies.[27]

Apropos of his comments, it occurred to me that impoverished Af-rican American patients on Medicaid, which, according to the trans-plant surgeon, reimburses 19 cents on the dollar, lack insurance that will cover immunosuppressive drugs; consequently, they are not eligi-ble for liver transplants. Thus, in the American medical system, the only power poor African American families possess is negative: They can say no and insist on continuing ICU care, hoping for a "miracle." They have no other power in a health-care system where they are denied some of the "miracles" offered to those who are more comfort-ably situated. In New Zealand, to the contrary, the number of liver transplants the Socialist government permits is limited (45 a year, for a population of 4 million). But the government pays for these trans-plants (a limited amount to cover all the expenses of the national New Zealand transplant unit) and for the subsequent immunosuppressive drugs. Thus, in New Zealand, fewer people receive transplants, but these are not limited by ability to pay.[28]

It is perhaps obvious that I prefer "fuzzy logic" based on moral discomfort to an attempt to quantify probabilities. No matter how many times one flips a coin, one cannot predict or influence the heads-tails-odds of the next toss. Too many American physicians still subscribe to Lord Kelvin's axiom, that whatever you know that cannot be expressed in numbers is "meagre and unsatisfactory."

Powerlessness to predict individual outcomes can lead to surgeons' classic justification of cheechee: "I've seen patients like this survive!" This is why, when it comes to decisions at the end of life, I believe that "moral discomfort" should trump statistical certainty—or uncer-tainty. It is also why surgeons should probably not make decisions about shifting from heroic to comfort care. If the heroic culture of American surgery does change, it will take a generation to do so. Until then, it might be wise to encourage surgeons to keep doing just what they have been selected and superbly trained to do: battle death to the bitter end.

Dying in an Academic American ICU: "Follow the Money"

"Science" is venerated in academic medical centers. The medical view of science, however, is often rather dated, with "facts" and "values" meticulously separated, a distinction contested by contemporary philosophers, historians, and sociologists of science.[29] When facts and values are alienated, with "hard" science that deals with "facts" valorized over "soft" science concerned with elusive subjects such as "values," then issues such as death and dying, which despite all efforts resist quantification, are perceived as messy, unattractive, and profoundly unscientific. Popular beliefs about male and female nature influence this evaluation: objectivity, reason, mind, and facts are cast as masculine; subjectivity, feeling, and nature are defined as feminine. Consequently, "soft" subjects such as death and dying are unreflectively identified as the natural province of nurses, social workers, and chaplains (who are perceived as somewhat feminine since they deal with "soft" spiritual matters).

In recent years, change has been evident. The theme for the 2001 meeting of the Society of Critical Care Medicine was "Blending Science and Compassion" and featured a series of presentations on "Compassionate End-of-Life Care in the Intensive Care Unit."[30] (Several speakers, however, commented on how small had been the previous audiences for talks on death and dying.) Another sign of change is indicated by the subject of the 2003 Brussels Consensus Meeting: "Challenges in End-of-Life Care in the ICU."[31]

Nevertheless, despite the fact that a number of highly intelligent and concerned intensivists are now working and publishing in this area[32]—funded in part by the Robert Wood Johnson Foundation[33]— the issue of compassionate care at the end of life is still perceived as unscientific, especially when compared with easily quantifiable "translational research" based on animal experiments or statistical manipulation of medico-genetic data.

Reflecting on how American intensivists deal with dying in the ICU, I was advised by an intensivist friend to "follow the money." It was obvious that research and publications on death and dying had been stimulated by the Robert Wood Johnson Foundation's Initiative on Death in America. This is neither unexpected nor corrupt. Research follows the money in every discipline, including my own field of anthropology. Few researchers can afford to fund their own investigations, and an investigator who did so would rank low in the academic prestige system as compared to a colleague with a generous grant from a private foundation or government agency.

"The money" is relatively simple in New Zealand. The Auckland ICU receives a fixed sum from the district health board, which covers salaries, equipment, supplies, and other identified costs. This is converted to an average hourly rate for each ICU patient, which is then billed to the appropriate hospital service (such as medicine or surgery). There is no fee for service system at all—nor is there any attempt to attribute specific costs, such as medicine or supplies, to individual patients. The rules regarding intensivists' salaries are even more transparent. The ICU has a 15-step salary scale based on years of service. Progression beyond Step 3 is based on an annual performance review; employees may be advanced more rapidly if their performance is rated as exceptional. (These reviews are conducted by intensivist colleagues and ICU personnel: senior nurses, residents, secretaries, and physiotherapists. I suspect such assessments, from colleagues and subordinates who spend most of their working time together, look very different from the top-down, "productivity"-focused reviews carried out in the Midwest Medical Center, which will be discussed below.)

The practices and regulations governing ICU reimbursement and intensivists' salaries in American academic medical centers are Byzantine. In some ways, they resemble the childhood game of Monopoly, where if you make a wrong step, you may be given a card saying "Do not pass go" or "Go immediately to jail."

The Midwest SICU makes no distinction between patients who can afford and those who cannot afford their services. (The New Zealand unit makes no distinction, as well, but in Auckland, neither the ICU nor the hospital receive less money for some patients and more for others.) Approximately 25 percent of the Midwest SICU patients are "self-pay," which in practice means either no pay or covered by Medicaid, which reimburses almost nothing for ICU care. Approximately 45 percent of the SICU patients are over age 65; the unit is reimbursed for these patients according to complex and constantly changing Medicare regulations. As the pool of older patients grows, with patient expectations and demands continually escalating, Medicare costs spiral while reimbursements are correspondingly cut. Reading the Medicare regulations is enough to give one a three-Tylenol headache. Definitions of what constitutes "critical care," and can consequently be reimbursed as such, bear little resemblance to what is actually done for patients in the ICU. Teaching residents is not reimbursed. Talking to families is reimbursed only under limited and very carefully defined circumstances: *"regular or periodic updates of the patient's condition, emotional support for the family, and answering questions regarding the patient's condition"* are specifically excluded (Italics mine). Documentation requirements for these regulations are extreme, with a mistake or choice of a wrong category leading to expenses being disallowed. Private insurers tend to follow the lead of Medicare, so that a Medicare regulation or refusal to reimburse may be echoed by BlueCross/BlueShield and other medical insurers. Consequently, following and documenting these complex requirements is expensive, consuming the time of doctors, secretaries, and personnel whose job it is to fit what actually occurs into these Procrustean categories. The hospitals have little input into these financial decisions; they are imposed from above. The behavior of intensivists, then, is influenced and often constrained by these regulations.

The processes that determine the salaries of the midwestern intensivists are correspondingly complex and opaque. Every year, the business office transmits information to the two ICU co-directors about the clinical work (involving patient care) carried out by each intensivist; this is expressed in terms of "relative value units" or RVUs (the scale Medicare uses to compare one doctor's workload with another's). The business office also provides a tally of grant funding for the year. The ICU co-directors evaluate the performance of each intensivist annually, computing the clinical dollars and grant dollars brought in, plus any special recognitions a doctor may have received; each co-director then gives salary and bonus recommendations to his superior, who forwards his recommendations to the chairman (of surgery for surgeons, and of anesthesiology for anesthesiologists).

The central fact, mentioned in my discussion of "no margin, no mission" (Chapter 9) is that every faculty member is expected to go out and generate revenue and at least try to cover his or her salary and expenses. Since money is tight, with ICU expenses rising and reimbursement shrinking, it is difficult to justify "uncompensated faculty time," which means time spent talking with families, building rapport, and teaching residents how to talk to families and make end-of-life decisions.

Consequently, in most academic ICUs in the United States—unless an ICU team has been specifically funded to study compassionate care at the end of life and devise innovations to improve it—communicating with families and helping patients to die "a good death" are not considered part of the *professional* responsibilities of critical care physicians. These responsibilities are *private;* their fulfillment depends on the ethical sensibilities of each intensivist. (As F. Scott Fitzgerald's Gatsby observed about his adored Daisy's love for her husband, it's "just personal.")[34] Because the processes of making compassionate decisions at the end of life and communicating well with families are defined as personal and optional, they are not imparted to residents as crucial techniques that should be mastered by every physician. (To repeat: Neither the practice nor the teaching of these are recompensed; they involve uncompensated faculty time.) In the Midwest SICU, I observed only one of the seven intensivists discuss these ethical and communication issues and teach residents how to make decisions and talk to families.[35] This man reported that he had become far more sensitized to end of life concerns after the death of his father. Here is an example of his teaching from my fieldnotes:

> Hunt [the intensivist] then talked . . . about what to do with a patient who has a terminal diagnosis yet is intubated [with a ventilator tube down his or her throat]. They've agreed ahead of time that there should be no heroic measures, yet family members find it hard to put the patient's desires ahead of their own. Family members often want to do everything possible because they can't bear to lose the patient, even when the patient might prefer to stop treatment. . . . She'll [the patient they're discussing during rounds] get a 40% response in six weeks [from more chemotherapy], but she can't breathe now. How does one balance cure against comfort? There's the personal decision: Do you want to continue therapy? Then there's the medical decision, which is separate: Is further therapy futile? The doctors must ask the right questions [of the family], said Hunt.

On the rare occasions when these subjects were broached during rounds, the residents listened with apparent interest. I suspect many residents want to learn how to handle death and dying with knowledge and empathy, how to demonstrate compassion and caring, how to communicate more effectively with families using plain English rather than medi-speak. Caring for people is why many young people go into medicine in the first place. During their training, however, young doctors are trained to transform patients' stories into cases, to "prioritize," dealing with technical matters before they devote time to emotional factors (if, indeed, they have time to devote), and to think about patients in the technical language valued by their superiors, a language that has no words or spaces for feelings.[36] The nurses were the ones who hugged patients and held their hands and who comforted distraught family members. The one critical care fellow who I observed treating family members of dying patients with warmth and compassion lacked "star quality," and he went to another hospital when his training was completed.

Handling death with consideration and care for patient and family was not spelled out as an explicit policy in the Midwest SICU. (If it were, the intensivists would have had to fight the surgeons every inch of the way, as no death is a "good death" for most surgeons—unless it happens to someone else's patient.) I heard no intensivist express pride in how well the unit handled dying or communicated with families; this was in striking contrast to the doctors' self-esteem regarding their technical expertise. As one intensivist declared to residents during rounds: "Our ICU, our school, our university is at the cutting edge of everything!" "The cutting edge" refers to knowledge of the latest findings in their field and expert deployment of the most advanced drugs and technology. Compassion and communication have no cutting edge: these old-fashioned medical virtues are either present or absent. The doctors were justifiably proud of the patients they saved who might have died in less-skilled ICUs, but no pride was expressed in what went on with patient and family when they lost someone. One of the SICU co-directors was interested in end-of-life issues; he talked compassionately and truthfully with families. He did not realize, however, how clearly his tone of voice and body language indicated discomfort and impatience to move on to the next task. I rarely observed the second co-director converse with family members, and he showed little apparent interest in or knowledge about the personal characteristics of patients and families. He delivered admirable, informed technical care but impressed me as somewhat uncaring.[37]

What the midwestern medical center intensivists lacked, which their New Zealand counterparts possessed, was *time*—time to talk, listen, reflect on ethical issues and families' emotional needs, time to discuss problems and perplexities with colleagues. It was a triumph that patients died as well as they did in the Midwest ICU, that families were informed as well as they in fact were; this occurred because the intensivists were decent and caring individuals. But, despite the hospital's slogan—"we care"—caring was not part of the SICU's institutional policy; it was exhibited by nurses, or by doctors as part of "uncompensated faculty time." (It is not surprising that in focus groups run by our research project, family members of ICU patients identified the nurse as the pivotal communicator and caregiver.)[38]

In other words, in academic medical center ICUs, not only are there *no* institutional mechanisms to encourage communication with families and compassionate (as well as technically accomplished) end–of–life care, there are *institutional constraints* against teaching and delivering such care. Hard-pressed critical care doctors, laboring to fulfill RVUs and write the grant proposals and conduct the research to bring in grant money, must employ their own uncompensated time to teach residents, answer questions, and provide emotional support for families. Unless they attract grant money for a demonstration project, CVUs (compassion value units) are neither prized, calculated, nor compensated by the institution—or by the government and private health-care funding agencies whose policies shape those of the financially stressed American medical centers.

A Heart of Wisdom

I have followed the money and come to a place I did not particularly want to reach. I had hoped to end with a discussion of how to oppose the "dominion of death," arguing that we cannot combat death by fighting it to the brutal end. Death always has the last word. A limitless battle against death leads only to human suffering, and social, cultural, and spiritual harm.[39] Death can have no dominion only when we realize that it is an essential part of life, that "though lovers be lost love shall not."

I planned to quote the Old Testament:

Teach us to number our days that we may get a heart of wisdom (Psalms 90: 12)

This would be followed by words of philosopher Hans Jonas, reflecting on the burden and blessing of mortality:[40]

It is a duty of civilization to combat premature death among humankind worldwide and in all its causes—hunger, diseases, war, and so on. As to your mortal condition as such, our understanding can have no quarrel about it with creation unless life itself is denied. As to each of us, the knowledge that we are here but briefly and a nonnegotiable limit is set to our expected time may even be necessary as the incentive to number our days and make them count.

Yes, but. . . .

All of these ways of combating the dominion of death are *individual*. Each of us must learn to number our days and make them count. Physicians must become more comfortable with the idea of death so they can support and nurture patients and families during this anguished process.[41] All of us—patients, families, and doctors—must accept the fact that death is not an unnatural event with failure to prevent it defined as therapeutic failure.[42]

But there is more to it. Providing compassionate ICU care for patients and families at the end of life is not entirely amenable to individual solutions; the problem is systemic or institutional.

We know some of the ways dying can be made less agonizing for patients and families, and we are constantly learning more. We have learned about drugs and techniques to assure comfort from the moment patients enter the ICU to the time they leave, whether that departure involves survival or death.[43] We are learning how to conduct conferences with families to inform them about the condition of the patient and to educate and support family members in helping them make difficult decisions about shifting from heroic to comfort care.[44] We know that families want more information than they generally receive from doctors[45] and that frequent updates help build a reservoir of trust that facilitates decision making at the end of life.[46] We know that young doctors must learn how to care for dying patients and talk to families. Some of us also realize:

> Efforts to provide a "good death" for patients and their families require close attention to not just their informational and decision-making needs, but also their emotional, spiritual and psychological needs.[47]

All of this takes *time*. And unless a medical center has a grant to study and devise innovative responses to these problems, time is exactly what today's hard-pressed ICU physicians do not have. They are busy racking up clinical RVUs (calculated in terms of activities compensated by Medicare), writing grant requests, and conducting research attempting to generate funds to cover their salaries and expenses.

One can call for an institutional commitment to these activities, but institutions, too, are hard-pressed. Academic medical centers, especially old, well-established ones, tend to be located in central city neighborhoods, with a high percentage of impoverished patients, who use the emergency room for their primary medical care and suffer from a disproportionate incidence of accidents and violence, with survivors often landing in the ICU. The ER, trauma department, and ICU costs for care of these patients are unreimbursed (or reimbursed by Medicaid at far less than the amounts that the institution expends to care for them). The costs, then, for uninsured patients or those "insured" by Medicaid, are borne by the institution—and eventually by all of us, who pay by being served by doctors who lack the time to talk to us and assuage our grief and uncertainty when a loved one is dying. We pay the price, as well, for unreasonable expectations, nurtured by media publicity, that encourage the fantasy that death is unnatural and can be postponed by technological advances. We also pay the price in the United States for regulations devised by legislators, and administered by bureaucrats, that deal with rising demands and unrealistic expectations by reducing or excluding reimbursement for teaching young doctors, comforting patients and families, and educating and supporting families as they make difficult decisions at the end of life.

Individual solutions, learning to number our days and accept death as part of life, will not eradicate these systemic problems. So long as American doctors and the media disseminate the notion that a technological fix will bring us closer to eternal life, we as a society will pay the price. So long as there are impoverished patients who cannot pay for medical care, all of us will pay the price. We, as a society, must follow the money—and put our money where our mouths are.

"Hard" Science, "Soft" Science, Social Science

The Anxiety of Methods

Fieldwork in ICUs

The reader unfamiliar with social scientific methods may want to know just what I did to learn what I learned. Social scientists may perhaps be interested in how I conduct research and my rationale for doing it this way.

I am following social scientific custom, placing this chapter on methods at the end. This is where the investigator discards any pretense of anonymity, revealing herself as a fallible human being with misgivings, mistakes, decisions, and dilemmas while conducting research. Medical articles, on the other hand, frequently begin with a brief summary, detailing the research context, objective, setting, subjects, measurements and main results, and conclusions.

I am neither a traditional social scientist writing theoretical jargon aimed primarily at colleagues, nor a medical researcher speaking primarily to physicians interested in how these findings may help them care for patients. I am writing for the educated reader—whether social scientist, layperson, or physician—someone who, perhaps by malignant chance rather than choice, has more to do with intensive care than he or she might wish. In this chapter, I give some notion of who I am, what I did in "the field," and how I conduct research. When reading an ethnography, I turn first to this section, as I am persuaded that anonymity in social research claims an indefensible objectivity. Since the fieldworker is her own measuring instrument, the reader needs to learn who made these particular observations and how she worked and lived.[1]

The method I use is called *fieldwork*, or *ethnographic research*. Sometimes described as "participant observation," this technique is employed by anthropologists, some sociologists, educational researchers, and others.[2] The term "ethnography" refers to a *method*, as well as to the *result*, a book based on the findings. Traditionally, fieldwork asks the researcher, as far as possible, to share the environment, problems, language, rituals, and social relations of a relatively bounded or delimited group of people.

Naturally, this sharing is limited. "Going native" even among the distant and exotic groups traditionally studied by anthropologists is usually more a fantasy of the researcher than an assessment shared by those studied. They know who you are. Anthropologists have married into the group;[3] others have spent 20 or 30 years studying the same community.[4] Such connections provide a unique perspective. Such familiarity, however, also causes problems: once *they* become *us*, loyalties and perceptions alter; the social scientist becomes a variety of "native observer,"[5] with a new set of interpersonal and ethical perplexities.[6]

As an ethnographer, you do have a role—especially if you have been studying the same group for more than a year. It is an odd role: You are, and yet are not, part of the group.

When conducting research, you cannot be invisible to doctors and nurses. They know who you are, whether or not you wear a white coat. Studying ICUs, sociologist Robert Zussman did not wear a lab coat; he felt this was "a type of deception entirely out of the spirit of notions of informed consent and patient rights."[7] I do wear one; it has convenient pockets to hold a pen, the index cards on which I write my notes, and various documents people give me; women's clothes rarely have pockets and I want my hands free to hold water, coffee, Kleenex, whatever.[8] Also, I then blend into the hospital milieu and am unlikely to be taken for an intrusive family member. On occasion, a family member will inquire about a patient; I always tell the questioner that I am an anthropologist studying the unit and direct that person to the resident or nurse who can answer their queries.

Some medical anthropologists and sociologists spend a good bit of time and effort attempting to master the scientific information they encounter.[9] Although I will ask a nurse or resident to explain a term that seems important, I make no special attempt to gain expertise.

Over time, I pick up enough to understand the gist of what is occurring. I am not focusing on *medicine* but on *people practicing medicine*. I have no fantasies of being a "little doctor"—I know the milieu, not the discipline.

Fieldwork differs in significant ways from quantitative hypothesis-based research. Rather than seeking to measure and predict, the fieldworker's primary aim is to understand. It is open ended; you enter "the field" to examine what is occurring, rather than clearly defining and delimiting exactly what will be investigated ahead of time.

Hypothesis-based research on social issues involving human interaction, employing rigorous validated instruments, can support or refute the initial hypothesis. By ignoring context and "irrelevant" variables, such research focuses narrowly on the phenomena being examined. Of course, values can creep in—in the unspoken assumptions that guide the ordering and phrasing of questions, and the choice of subjects to whom the instrument will be presented. Values may also enter, as many researchers realize, in the difference between those who choose to respond to a questionnaire and those who refuse to do so.

But in the end, however well designed and scrupulously administered, such research cannot surprise the investigator. The hypothesis is supported or disconfirmed; the fact that the truly interesting, influential phenomena were not addressed by the instrument, if this is indeed so, is not indicated. These phenomena remain undiscovered. Context and complex ambiguous interactions are just "noise" interfering with the inquiry. The more rigorous the investigation, the less the complexity of human motives and interaction are taken into account.

This is an effective type of research, when using mice in the laboratory to study sepsis, manipulating rats to discover the most effective way to preserve the liver, or testing the efficacy of various drugs or treatments. The intentions of the animals or the patients, their social interactions, if any, are irrelevant. These must be filtered out behaviorally or, if necessary, through research design.

Such methods have distinct limitations, however, when dealing with human interaction. The investigator can find out little that was not covered by the original hypothesis.

As a fieldworker, I "hang out" with the people I am studying, observing what occurs, and recording whatever catches my attention. This can be anxiety-producing; you do not have a clear pre-planned map of just what you are going to do, and when you are going to do it.[10] Charles Bosk, who studied surgical residents, notes that he feels "a sense of respect for data-collecting procedures which allow the researcher to keep the sensuous world at a distance, and which thereby allow him to avoid the self-exposure, self-reflection, and self-doubt endemic to fieldworkers."[11]

Conducting fieldwork, I often feel somewhat apprehensive: Am I in the right spot? Did I stay there long enough? What am I missing? After more than 34 years of doing this, however, I reassure myself with the fact that, no matter how much I have missed—and there is no doubt that I miss a great deal—each time I have carried out a study, I managed to learn enough to understand and describe what was observed.[12]

Ethnographic research is generally more prolonged than a quantitative study. Although you have some idea of what you are interested in, you cannot specify in advance the exact nature of what will be examined, analyzed, and compared. Rather than entering the situation with pre-planned and possibly arbitrary measures and criteria, your research is guided by unfolding events and discoveries. To give just one example: When I first started studying the Midwest SICU, I observed conflict between the surgeons and intensive care physicians who shared responsibility for patients. I decided to spend time with several surgeons who sent patients to the unit to observe their relations with their patients and with the ICU attending physicians. This was not planned beforehand; it emerged from my observations, leading to further observations and formulations about conflicting moral economies.

Because it is not limited by predefined procedures and events to be examined, ethnographic research is extremely flexible; it can adapt to unforeseen and rapidly changing circumstances. Such research is relatively time- and effort-consuming, however, because the research route has not been precisely mapped in advance.

When conducting fieldwork in an ICU, I generally attend morning rounds; afterward, I'll stroll around the unit observing what is going on; stand in one place for a while surveying the action; spend an hour or two following a resident, fellow, or nurse; or spend an entire day observing an ICU attending physician at work. I take brief notes on 3×5 index cards stashed in the pocket of my white coat. Residents sometimes express interest in what I am writing, and I then display the card, which contains briefly scribbled phrases and quotations. (As Zussman noted in a similar situation, the willingness to display one's notes seems to allay any fears.)[13]

That evening, or the following day, I type the fieldnotes on my home computer. The brief scribbled notes act as mnemonics, helping me remember just what occurred and how I reacted to it.[14] Although my hanging out in the ICU may appear somewhat casual, the subsequent transcription, amplification, coding, and analysis of the fieldnotes are highly structured processes.

For coding fieldnotes, I use a computer program designed for ethnographic research.[15] I devise the codes, which can be people's names, ideas, concepts. I can then use the program to retrieve every instance of an observation on a particular subject: For example, I can call up and compare every example of "teaching" in my fieldnotes.

I transcribe, code, and analyze my notes at home, not at my office in the hospital. *I want no one to have access to my fieldnotes.* The risks and benefits of ethnographic research differ from those posed by biomedical research.[16] Fieldwork risks breaching confidentiality, which can injure or upset those studied; the benefits are more general than those of medical research, being primarily to knowledge and, if one is fortunate, to improving practices in a particular milieu or profession.

The method is labor- and time-intensive—it takes as much time for me to write up and code material as to conduct the original observations. The results, however, can be productive. As an "interpretive science,"[17] ethnography—when dealing with familiar rather than exotic settings—can be judged in part by the shock of recognition, the feeling that "yes, that's the way it is! I never thought of it that way before."

Ethnographic research observes people in action, over time, as events unfold; consequently, the findings are richer than verbal responses to an interview or closed-ended survey,[18] in which subjects may tell the interviewer what they think she wants to hear, or what they think they are doing, or how they think they might behave in a hypothetical situation—all of which may differ significantly from observed behavior. Naturally, bias may affect results. (Bias affects survey research as well, where responses are shaped by the questions asked and the way in which they are phrased, as well as by the questions *not* asked.)

The Anxiety of Method

If there is one point of consensus among sociologists concerning field methods, it is this: the sociologist is there to study a social scene and not to change it, so whenever possible, do not interfere.[19]

Sociologists tend to be much concerned with methods. Anthropologists have written about methods,[20] but as a group, we are generally more relaxed than sociologists and less impressed by what is frequently presented as *the scientific paradigm:* Do not interfere with, and thus alter, the social scene under observation.

The history of the two disciplines may affect the level of methodological anxiety. Sociologists traditionally studied their own societies, where their activity could be observed by others. In addition, sociology has as ancestors, Comte, the father of positivism, who pictured the natural sciences as branches with sociology at the summit, with the ability to explain the phenomena uncovered by the subordinate branches,[21] and Durkheim, who advocated conceptualizing social facts [*faits sociaux*] as "things" [*choses*] to be objectively studied, classified, and measured, apart from their individual occurrences.[22]

The anthropological "ancestors," on the other hand, were less concerned about the methodological purity of their data. Consider the Victorian anthropologist J. G. Frazer, about whom the story is told that when asked about natives he had known responded "But heaven forbid!"[23] A British gentleman might write about "savages" but he did not associate with them. Then, think of Malinowski, whose idyllic picture of being set down by himself on a tropical isle,

> paddling on the lagoon, watching the natives under the blazing sun at their garden work, following them through the patches of jungle and on the winding beaches and reefs . . .[24]

was challenged by the posthumous publication of his diaries.[25] Finally, contemplate Evans-Pritchard, who wrote an anthropological classic, *The Nuer*, based on intermittent, somewhat limited, visits to a group being "pacified" by military means during his study.[26] Few readers were in a position to check the methods or findings of the early anthropological studies of exotic peoples.

A Personal Note on Research Methods

As a graduate student in psychology in the mid-1960s, I was disturbed by my course in experimental psychology. The young professor kept teaching the class *how* (how to identify and construct a "parsimonious," "elegant," "scientific" experiment) while I kept trying to inquire *why* (why take all the trouble to do this?). At the time, I lacked the language and knowledge to formulate my gut reaction to her teachings, and she was too newly hatched from graduate school to understand my objections. It seemed to me (had I but words to express it) that the more elegant and well-designed an experiment, the less it had to do with actual human beings relating to one another in the "booming buzzing confusion" of real life. After obtaining an M.A. in psychology, I switched with relief to a graduate program in anthropology, which promised to deal with human interaction in real life and real time.

As an anthropology graduate student, however, I encountered an interesting phenomenon. Those professors, and authorities assigned as course reading, who advocated "rigorous," "formal," "scientific" methods disdained their colleagues who conducted "sloppy," "unscientific" research, whose writings were dismissed as a species of literature. The mantle of Science seemed to confer an unquestioned intellectual—and moral—superiority on those who assumed it.

After receiving a Ph.D in 1975, it took me a long time to find my "voice." Eventually, I rejected my advisor's advice to write in the passive voice; it surely *sounded* more scientific, but was far duller. I also jettisoned the fly-on-the-wall fantasy of the social scientist as a transparent unseen observer, who did her best not to influence the actions she was observing. *Of course* my presence influenced what went on. How could it not? Attempting not to influence what went on (whether in a rural Jamaican village or a feminist consciousness-raising group), pretending not to influence it, writing as though what occurred was not thereby affected, began to seem rather like Winnie-the-Pooh, rising skyward holding a balloon, hoping he looked like a black cloud rather than a bear with a balloon seeking honey. If this were "science" I wanted none of it. I began to wonder about the hierarchy of impersonality that endows some researchers with the moral and intellectual hauteur to look down on others.

What Makes an Inquiry Scientific?

Is science a search for knowledge or understanding? Or is it defined by methodology, or methodologies—the more "objective," "value free," or "impersonal," the more "scientific? Is science defined by how you seek? What you find? Who you are?[27]

I begin with a simple question: If the celebrated physicist Heisenberg determined that, even in physics, observing something alters whatever is being observed, why all the fuss about "objectivity" and hands-off observation? And, if facts and values cannot, in truth, be disentangled,[28] what does "value-free" research consist of?

Philosophers, historians, and sociologists of science have challenged allegedly value-neutral scientific research, showing how cultural factors influence findings and formulations in the natural, medical, and social sciences.[29] Some, but not all of these critics are feminists. Evelyn Fox Keller, who began as a physicist, observes:

> Careful attention to what questions get asked, of how research programs come to be legitimated and supported, of how theoretical disputes are resolved, of "how experiments end" reveals the working of cultural and social norms at every stage.[30]

Keller indicates the ways in which the conventional accounts scientists offer of their successes, as well as their descriptions of the "laws of nature," are rooted in metaphor, which is by no means culture- or value-free.[31]

If such post-Kuhnian inquiry is convincing[32]—and I, for one, find it so—then why does the objectivity/impersonality/value-free hierarchy still exist? Why is "hard" science considered superior to "soft"?

Keller argues that the language, tacit presuppositions, expectations, and assumptions shared by natural (or "hard") scientific researchers—which include the assumption that scientific language is transparent and neutral and, therefore, does not require examination—encourages the reliance on shared conventions and metaphors, which are inevitably culture based.[33]

Something else is going on, as a number of feminist scholars have indicated. Popular beliefs, or "myths," about male and female nature influence the hierarchy of scientific value. As noted in chapter 10, a series of cultural dichotomies cast objectivity, reason, and mind as masculine, while subjectivity, feeling, and nature, are perceived as feminine.[34] In this tacit division—between public and private, impersonal and personal, masculine and feminine—the masculine polarity is valorized. Consequently, in a barely disguised (tautological) phallic metaphor, "hard" science is more scientific than "soft."

This anxiety of method—who wants to be defined as soft?—extends beyond the social sciences. In medicine, surgery is more valorized, more masculine, more "scientific"—even when conducted by women—than psychiatry,[35] while biologically based psychiatrists disdain their "softer" colleagues, who converse with patients rather than treat them with drugs.[36] Academic surgeons, who conduct scientific research (preferably "hard," "bench" research), look down on those in private practice. And in critical care medicine, until recently, the investigation of compassionate end-of-life care was slighted by those interested in "harder" more "scientific" issues. Even when the topic became intellectually acceptable, researchers attempted to apply rigorous, objective, value-free methods, as though these would help erase the stigma of subjectivity.

Applying Objective Methods to a Subjective Issue

Many biomedically based research articles on end-of-life issues in the ICU miss the mark. Some are admonitory, exhorting doctors to do or avoid various behaviors. Others offer basic principles, such as "benevolence" or "autonomy," with little guidance in applying these principles in the day-by-day, hour-by-hour care of gravely ill patients, who are often so sick (in addition to being intubated[37] and highly sedated) that a term such as "autonomy" has little relevance to their situation.[38] Some research programs make such drastic errors in understanding the social structure of medicine, in taking into account the on-the-ground dynamics of doctor–nurse interaction, that they make egregious social mistakes (e.g., in who should tell what to whom) nullifying their expensive efforts at improving practice.[39] "Validated instruments" are apparently more highly regarded than perceptive researchers; the medium, the objective value-free qualities of the methodology, becomes more important than those who utilize it. There seems to be an almost automatic assumption that if the tools are sufficiently "scientific," almost anyone can brandish them and get good results. This, as any surgeon will tell you, is nonsense.

Another problem undermines some medical research efforts:

> The physician is accustomed to a leadership role, regardless of knowledge base. Physicians tend to take it for granted that they know more than anyone else about subjects related to medicine; the more senior the physician, the more confident he (or she) is, of his or her knowledge base.[40]

When this certitude is linked to a difficulty many physicians exhibit in *listening* rather than holding forth,[41] we find studies where the senior physician-researchers are unable to attend to, and consequently learn from nonmedical colleagues and, more important, from the people they are purportedly studying. The ability to listen is as crucial in studying human interaction as it is in conducting effective end-of-life discussions;[42] one must be able listen to *silences* as well as words, to attend to what people are *not* saying as well as what they say.[43] This overconfidence and underreceptiveness, added to an excessive reliance on method rather than theoretical insight and creative imagination, can lead to self-fulfilling prophecies, or a kind of routine-journeyman application of instruments to groups, as though such mechanical procedures will inevitably produce significant results.

Let me emphasize that I am not condemning all biomedical writings on end-of-life issues. Some are outstanding.[44] But a number of research reports seem, somehow, off-kilter; one knows little more after reading them than before.

Perturbing the System

Some years ago, I was on a panel where a medical anthropologist, prominent in a program on medical ethics, described how, when conducting research in a hospital, she kept silent when observing unethical and, on occasion, dangerous behavior by medical personnel. She said she did not want to ruin her "rapport" with the staff. I was appalled. Not only was her stance profoundly unethical, I was not at all sure it was methodologically sound. Is it truly necessary and/or scientific to conceal who you are, what you feel, your own values and reactions, while trying to elicit those of the people you are studying? Is it really more scientific to try to avoid influencing what goes on, pretending that your presence has little or no effect on those you study?

Sociologist Renée Ansbach, in her superb study of a neonatal ICU, describes, with a twinge of what almost sounds like regret, how once she did intervene.[45] She deliberately asked a question that led a resident to formulate a treatment plan for a neonate with a dismal prognosis in a situation where the doctors had been postponing making a difficult decision. Nevertheless, in another section of her methodological appendix, Ansbach wonders "why a detached stance toward research subjects should necessarily be considered 'objective' or 'free of bias.'"[46] (One gets the impression that Ansbach is, at best, somewhat ambivalent about the detached stance her mentors may well have recommended.) She explains why and how she did not get co-opted when she adopted a more participatory style in her second research site, mentioning her attempt to avoid the "Hawthorne effect."[47] In his study of intensive care units, Robert Zussman is anxious about pretending to be a doctor, as though wearing a white coat would deceive any of the residents, nurses, and attendings with whom he interacted.[48] But why work so hard to avoid the Hawthorne effect if the Heisenberg effect still holds?

I do not expect to sway those investigators who suffer from what has been characterized as "physics envy" (incorrectly, considering Heisenberg's indeterminacy principle). But other ways to conduct social research do exist.[49]

Rather than pretending to herself and her audience that she is utterly neutral, objective, and value-free—a state that is, in point of fact, almost impossible to achieve—the researcher can join in. Participant observation is the anthropological method, par excellence, and the observing social scientist can participate in whatever is going on as much as possible.[50] If you are there for some time, as a living, reacting fellow human being, rather than a human pretending to be a disembodied fly-on-the-wall, the people you are studying will create a space for you. In the early 1980s, after almost 18 months of studying surgeons at the same hospital, I took part in a festive dinner attended by surgeons from several local hospitals; we went around the long table, introducing ourselves: "I'm Joan Cassell, I'm the anthropologist who studies them," I announced, as "my" surgeons smiled possessively. Although most of these men had not wanted me at their hospital and had done their best to frustrate my investigations, by this time, I was *their* anthropologist. You are still an outsider, but a highly privileged outsider, to whom people reveal confidences or recount their side of a dispute when they suspect you have heard their antagonist's version.

One reason anthropologists may be less apprehensive about interacting freely with the host people is that, when conducting research in distant sites, we frequently bring our families with us.[51] A young child cannot be taught to be reticent, objective, or value-free in the field. Children interact and, as a parent, you too interact, frequently with quite a bit of emotion. One of the things you learn, with children in the field, is that such open and unguarded interaction brings rich rewards in the form of data. When you and your children perturb the system, you learn things you would discover no other way.

Children are not necessary in order to perturb the system. The researcher's words, actions, and interactions can elicit actions and reactions from the people studied. Neutrally inquiring "Why did you (he, or they) do that?" does not necessarily bring more or better data than asking "Why in the world did you (he, or they) ever do *that?*" Thus, when I told the women surgeons I was studying that they needed the kind of doctor's wife I had been for almost 30 years, several then spoke of the difficulties of *not* having someone to assume the emotional, social, and on occasion physical responsibilities of daily life.[52]

As a researcher, I no longer even attempt to be objective or invisible. I react to what goes on: I agree with some statements, disagree with others, am upset by some actions, delighted by others, disapprove of some people, admire others. This does not mean that I cast myself as a central figure in what goes on in the SICUs I study. I am an observer, very much on the sidelines. But I am by no means neutral or value-free. I say what I think; I do not proclaim it, nor do I interrupt the flow of activities. But I have, on occasion, interjected a comment during patient rounds, pointing out, for example, that behavior by a family characterized as "difficult," might be related to social class, and that attempting to gain the family's trust by listening to their concerns could save time and trouble in caring for that patient. Other times, I have quietly complimented someone for defending a course of action or viewpoint I supported.

It has taken me many years of conducting fieldwork and gaining confidence in myself and my own way of doing things to be able to be so open. I believe this openness has allowed me to collect data that I would never have been given access to otherwise. When I react as a living, breathing human being, with ideas, opinions, and even prejudices of my own, others react to me in a similar fashion. (Some of the material in this book could not have been collected by a "fly on the wall.")

Naturally, in polarized field situations, and most situations contain contending factions and viewpoints, the researcher tends to view happenings through the lens of those individuals she finds most sympathetic. But if she can manage to spend time with people belonging to more than one group or faction, she may experience the "Rashomon effect" of the same occurrences viewed from such differing perspectives that "reality" becomes fractured, the issue then becoming *whose* reality.[53] Thus, when I spend time with the surgeons who send patients to the SICU I spent the most time observing, I am immersed in an utterly different set of concerns, viewpoints, and ethical relationships than when I am with the critical care doctors. When the two groups disagree about patient management, it is no longer a question of which is the "*real*" reality, of who has right on his or her side, so much as a demonstration of utterly divergent epistemologies or moral economies.

Highly participatory research has pitfalls. The researcher can become what some Marxists would disapprovingly describe as "co-opted."[54] Let me note that those social scientists who accuse colleagues who express favorable sentiments toward doctors of being co-opted, do not necessarily conduct objective research, themselves. Their supposedly value-free investigations frequently depict physicians as venal, collusive in hiding misbehavior, contemptuous of patients, and falsely omniscient.[55]

Nevertheless, the question arises: When studying a powerful profession such as medicine, am *I* "co-opted?" As an ethnographer, I surely sympathize with many of the people I study, and I tend, while studying them, to perceive reality through their eyes. In this respect, my data-collection and -processing techniques are helpful. I scribble brief notes in the field, while participating as much as someone—who knows a good bit about doctors but little about medicine—can. Amplifying them at home that evening or the next day puts a certain distance between me and what occurred. Coding the notes adds a second degree of emotional distance. When comparing various instances of a coded occurrence, I perceive differences and similarities; this comparison generates insight about occurrences, leading to additional categories, or several categories being combined as a larger class. Writing up my findings, creates a third degree of distancing. No longer involved with the individuals and activities, I can reinterpret occurrences, placing an observation or observations in a still more inclusive category, or entirely altering my interpretation of what went on. Co-optation attenuates as, drawing back to view a larger picture, I perceive the ways in which I may have been manipulated, or have manipulated myself, into a sympathy or position I no longer hold. (Moreover, since I attempt to view what occurs through the eyes of different participants: nurses, residents, intensivists, surgeons, and, to some extent patients and their families, I get a somewhat varied, or Rashomon-like, perspective that makes it more difficult to be co-opted by one particular group.)

Immersing yourself in the system, having strong feelings about places, people, behavior, can help give you an insider's knowledge of that system. No, you are not a native, a true insider, but to the extent to which you engage with those studied and enter the system to the best of your ability, you learn about that system, the way it works and does not work, what affects it, which individuals facilitate its workings, and which ones, in contrast, gum up the works.

Describing the System: The Ethnographic Monograph

When an ethnographic researcher enters the system, the first thing to consider is the degree of participation. The second is the subsequent description of that participation. In recent years, anthropologists, who have rejected the disembodied fly-on-the-wall fantasy, have turned to *embodied* descriptions of their research.[56]

It is a matter of taste and temperament. Some will denigrate such unabashedly subjective, highly participatory accounts as mere "literature," "memoir," or postmodern pretentiousness. Others will find such "narrative ethnography"[57] more interesting, involving, and communicative of what actually occurs in an alien social setting than the "flat, neutral, and 'sludgy'" writing frequently presented as objective, value-free social scientific discourse.[58]

It is obvious that I am one of those who writes herself into what occurred. I was there. I reacted. I do not pretend otherwise. Whenever possible, I try to bring the reader to the research site with me, perhaps to see what I saw, to feel what I felt, or if I've given enough detail, perhaps to take strong exception to my position and conclusions.

The narrative turn—which is perhaps more a narrative *return*—has even moved to the outskirts of medicine, affecting psychoanalysis,[59] medical ethics,[60] and medical anthropology.[61] From the Scriptures to the Mahabharata to American Indian origin myths, stories have always been a way of teaching, informing, enlightening. Sociologist Arthur Frank speaks of "thinking with stories," a powerful phrase for a powerful process in which narrative knowledge of a person's story can lead to morally informed professional decisions.[62]

In the end, I write the kind of books I enjoy reading. Rather than presenting complex theoretical formulations, I often employ "an argument of images."[63] Some readers may share my narrative predilection; others may find my approach soft-headed. Is what I do "science"? Well, to tell the truth, I do not care: I prize insight and understanding more than the benison of "science." But then again, I might be more of a scientist than I realize.

Notes

Introduction

1. van Gennep 1960; Turner 1967.

2. The rationale for the change was that motor vehicle "accidents" are rarely *completely* accidental; the behavior of the driver is often implicated.

3. DiGiacomo (1987) quotes Susan Sontag discussing her own cancer: "Illness is the night-side of life, a more onerous citizenship. Everyone who is born holds dual citizenship, in the kingdom of the well and in the kingdom of the sick" (Sontag 1978: 3). Also see Arthur Frank 1995.

4. Cassell 1991a, 1998.

5. National Institute of Nursing Research grant NRO5124.

6. Cassell 1980, 1981, 1982a, 1982b, 1991; Wax and Cassell, eds. 1979; Cassell and Wax, eds. 1980; Cassell and Jacobs, eds. 1987.

7. Various bills have been introduced, but so far not ratified, declaring that data from projects financed by government agencies belong to the government and must be submitted when demanded. Interestingly, strict regulations have been passed on protecting patient privacy. So far as I know, the possible contradictions between these two approaches have not been discussed.

8. 1984; Benner and Wrubel 1989.

9. Eric Cassell noted that the distinction between disease and illness is paralleled by a distinction between curing and healing. Killing bacteria, bringing down fever, and enabling a patient with pneumonia to breathe, will cure the *disease;* but there are other aspects of the *illness*—the patient's fear, isolation from family and friends, and painful dependence on other people—that must be addressed in order to restore well-being (1976: 16).

10. 1995: 3–4.

11. 1946: 54.

12. Lock 2001; Daston 1995.

13. Payer 1996: 129.

14. 1996: 121.

15. See Lock 2001: 488; Crippen et al. 2002. Daston says her use of the phrase "moral economy" is not indebted to its original use by E. P. Thompson (1991).

16. I could employ the phrase of W. I. Thomas 1966, contending that the

191

parties hold incompatible *definitions of the situation* in which they are acting, or follow Weber 1946, and discuss the ethic [*Ethik*] characterizing a particular vocation or religious group. I use the term "ethic," but it does not quite encompass the depth and breadth of the phenomenon I am attempting to describe. Alternatively, I might emulate Bateson 1936 or Redfield 1955 who speak of *ethos* as compared with *eidos*.

17. I have altered as many details as possible, and both physicians have reviewed this account to make sure I did not violate the doctors' or patient's confidentiality.

18. Bi-pap is a form of mechanical ventilation using a mask, which does not require a tube or a tracheotomy.

19. They removed the fluid.

20. Liquid in the lungs.

21. The tube attached to the ventilator removed.

Chapter One

1. A tracheotomy, or "trach," is an opening through the front of the neck into the trachea (windpipe). A tube is inserted, permitting the attachment of a mechanical ventilator to assist breathing. A "perc trach," or percutaneous tracheotomy, is performed at the bedside; a surgical tracheotomy is generally done in the OR. (The term "tracheotomy" shortened to "trach" is used in the United States, while New Zealand and Britain use "trachestomy" or "trachee.")

2. The nurse injected the patient with a neuromuscular blocker; this blocks all the nerves in the body so that the patient is unable to move. This medication is supposed to be administered or authorized by a physician, but in this emergency situation, the nurse had to act fast and obtain retrospective authorization.

3. Nurses are supposed to wait for doctors' orders before carrying out such procedures, but if it was not mentioned on the patient's chart, it theoretically did not occur.

4. "Bagging" is artificial breathing by manually squeezing a bag containing oxygen that is connected to the patient's airway. It is performed by the nurse or physician.

5. Fentanyl is a narcotic pain reliever similar to morphine; it acts faster, however, and does not last as long.

6. Mackay 1993: 43–44.

7. I had been carrying out participant observation in the SICU for six months, long enough to have learned that most patients who came to the unit with gunshot wounds had been shot by "unknown assailants." Or, as one cynical resident worded it: "I was just leaving the university with my mother when some dude came up and shot me!"

8. Redfield 1953: 20–22; also see E. J. Cassell 1974, who first applied the concept in the medical arena.

9. See Wax and Ray 2002.

10. See, for example, Gilligan 1982; Chodorow 1978; Noddings 1984; Belenky, Clinchy, Goldberger, and Tarule 1986.

11. Let me emphasize that I am not saying that morality is assigned to women,

but that Redfield's concept of the moral order, emphasizing face-to-face bonds between people, is in our culture most frequently conceptualized as "the woman's way."

12. Chiarella 2002: 39–55.

13. In 2001, the SICU had 5 male and 55 female nurses; in 2002, there were 10 male and 62 female nurses.

14. Chambliss 1996: 80–84.

15. This occurred in a medical center whose slogan, on every wall throughout the hospital, was "We care." Describing these mishaps, the distraught daughter said of the authorities whose attention to slogans and inattention to caring permitted such errors: "They don't get it. They just don't get it!"

16. 1996: 63.

17. Benner and Wrubel 1989.

18. Critical care nurse Lynn Schallom.

19. Hindwood 1991, cited by Chiarella 2002: 53.

20. Chiarella 2002: 53.

21. A resident who worked with my former husband at Bellevue Hospital in the 1950s had a stock answer for people who inquired, "How can I ever thank you?" He would respond: "Ever since the Phoenicians invented money, there's one universally accepted way."

22. Temporary nurses can be hired by the day from agencies that specialize in this. The agencies charge far more than full-time nurses earn (I was quoted $50 a day as opposed to $24 for an experienced nurse). Moreover, agency nurses do not know the routine of wherever they are sent: where drugs and devices are kept, what drugs are favored in this particular unit, or how this particular unit and hospital do things.

23. Wolfe 1987.

24. Shepherd 1993.

25. Chambliss 1996.

26. Chiarella 2002. Her data come primarily from Australia, but she also discusses England, Canada, and the United States.

27. The nurse whose responsibility was to see that staffing was adequate.

28. Chambliss 1996: 75–76.

29. See Fitzgerald 2001.

30. Patients are placed on isolation status to protect them, or others, from contamination by highly infectious organisms. Before medical personnel and family members enter the room, they are supposed to don gloves and gowns.

31. Cluff and Binstock, eds. 2001.

32. Ludmerer and Fox, 2001: 131.

Chapter Two

1. The number of residents was not fixed, but six or seven were usually assigned to the (then) 18-bed unit. The unit has subsequently expanded to 24 beds, while the number of residents has decreased.

2. Today, residents are formally described by the number of years since they graduated from medical school: PGY1 (postgraduate year one, who used to be

called an "intern" and is still informally called so), PGY2, PGY3, etc. I suspect the term "house officer" is left from the days when residents were expected to live in the hospital.

3. I was told that the situation reversed in 2003. Anesthesiology skims off the "cream," while surgery programs have difficulties filling their slots. This means surgery programs are less selective and the residents, as a group, weaker.

4. Let me note here that this refers *only* to the few residents I encountered in the SICU who had completed medical school and residency in Asia and practiced medicine there before being recruited to the anesthesia residency program at the Midwest medical center. I was told that other residents, with similar training and background, were superior. And this surely does *not* apply to the American-born and the American-trained Asian doctors I encountered; some of these young doctors were excellent.

5. When I first began studying surgeons, I could not understand why attendings frequently ridiculed neophytes in public; I finally realized it was a long-established method of instruction, which I thought of as "teaching by humiliation" (Bosk 1979).

6. The pupils did not react to light, which indicates severe neurological damage probably prefiguring death.

7. The patient was near moribund.

8. An intern who was there when the patient arrived commented: "It's the most disgusting thing I've ever seen!" He reported that the patient was given 26 units of blood, plus plasma (which is similar to blood), and it was utterly pointless. Blood was pouring out of the bed as they were putting it into her. A cynical nurse said "Why don't we just hook her up" (so the liquid that was pouring out could just be put back into her). He did not know how much of the hospital's resources were wasted. "It was really bizarre," he commented. When I asked this surgical intern why he thinks the surgeon did this, he said, "It's a shameful thing. It's better to have the patient die in the ICU than in the OR." In other words, the surgeon feels shame when the patient dies on his watch. See Buchman, Cassell, Wax, and Ray 2002.

9. Gordon 1988: 279.

10. Daston 1995: 10.

11. In some academic centers, these physicians are contemptuously referred to as LMDs, defined by Konner (1988: 385) as "Local Medical Doctor; the patient's town or neighborhood physician; usually condescending; often frankly derogatory." To be fair, I never heard this term used at the Midwest medical center and I, suspect that a young doctor who used it in the SICU would be reproved.

12. The term "n" represents the number of participants in an experiment.

13. Kelvin 1904.

14. Shaw (2003: 39–53), who studied genetic clinics, contrasts the diagnostic expertise of skilled clinicians, based on an intuitive "gut feeling" backed by years of hands-on experience, as opposed to junior physicians' reliance on molecular tests.

15. Bosk 1979.

16. Cassell 1991a: 9–32.

17. Weber 1946: 155.

18. Daston 1995: 5. Daston continues: "This is a psychology at the level of whole cultures, or at least subcultures, one that takes root within and is shaped by quite particular historical circumstances."

19. Thernstrom 1994; Cluff and Binstock 2001.

20. This punishing schedule was subsequently ameliorated as I go on to describe.

21. Until 2003, the Midwest surgical residents spent five clinical years, with a similar grueling schedule, and from two to four years conducting basic laboratory research. This prepared them to be "academic surgeons," teaching, conducting research, and operating. The Texas program, which prepares "practicing" as opposed to "academic" surgeons, omitted the lab years.

22. One woman surgeon responded that she is convinced that surgery can be imparted in 80 hours a week and believes that abusive work and hours should be eliminated. She noted, however, that with the new regulations, senior surgeons are wasting time "counting hours"; and she believes that the rigidity of the new rules, with no room for give and take, will definitely compromise resident training.

23. Sargant 1957.

24. Bosk 1979; Buchman et al. 2002.

25. The New Zealand registrars came from training programs in critical care (which is a separate specialty with its own residency programs in New Zealand), surgery, emergency medicine, anesthesia, and internal medicine.

26. The Texas residents came from training programs in surgery, orthopedics, rehabilitation medicine, and anesthesiology. First- and second-year residents spent approximately a month in the unit. They were supervised by two third-year surgery residents, who took responsibility for teaching, responding to emergencies, and conducting end-of-life discussions with families.

27. William Nolen, who was at Bellevue at the same time, discusses his experiences with similar zest (Nolen, 1950). Although the value of the dollar has changed enormously since the 1950s, I suspect the $35,000 annual salary of today's residents is more generous than the 1950s salaries, which assumed that residents were unmarried and living at the hospital (which was rarely the case).

28. President's message, Connections 2001, 2002.

29. A documentary filmmaker who filmed a series on the history of baseball.

30. Nolen's epigraph to the book about his Bellevue residency (1950) expresses this: "My father was a lawyer. When I was a boy he often said to me, 'Billy, if you're smart, when you grow up you'll be a doctor. Those bastards have it made.' I took my father's advice, and I dedicate this book to his memory."

31. I remember a party, when my former husband was a fellow in infectious disease, where all the young doctors went out of their way to be kind to the husband of a microbiologist researcher who worked in an adjacent lab; the husband described himself as a lawyer who had gotten into the movie business by accident. He was a quiet man, some years older than his wife, who serenely endured being patronized by a roomful of young doctors. Reading the *New York Times* the next morning, I discovered that this man was the president of one of the most successful film companies in the country.

32. Ludmerer (1999: 93) says of the "pre-match" days: "Many teaching hospitals would pressure students to commit to their program before a competing

teaching hospital had made its appointments. This led to a major dilemma for students: to accept a position at a less desirable hospital, or wait to hear from a more desirable hospital, risking the chance of ending up with no appointment at all."

33. On "learning in practice" see Lave and Wenger 1991.

34. Ludmerer 1999: 96.

35. Theoretically, the residents were unmarried, although Nolen points out that among the seven interns in his cadre, all single, five were married by the end of the first year. He notes that when he started at Bellevue, interns made $65 a month plus room and board at the hospital, while as a Chief Resident he made $190 a month, and that the long hours with low pay was hard on wives. He asserts: "We were all in debt, or getting by with the help of handouts from parents or in-laws" (1950: 151).

36. Ludmerer 1999: 96–98.

37. 1999: 59.

Chapter Three

1. An "outstanding" woman must surmount a number of double-binds to be recognized as such. High visibility can be labeled "pushiness" by superiors and "bitchiness" by nurses, while low visibility may cruise below the radar screen. See Cassell 1998.

2. The specialty is so new that many ICUs in smaller hospitals are still run by physicians who have not completed fellowships or passed critical care boards.

3. For certification as a medical intensivist, the candidate must finish a three-year residency in internal medicine and then a three-year fellowship in pulmonary medicine. The standards vary in different countries. In France, for example, completing a residency in internal medicine automatically classifies the physician as an intensivist (although other routes exist, as well), while in New Zealand and Australia, critical care is a separate specialty with its own residency program, preparing the graduate to conduct medical and surgical intensive care.

4. Clinical acumen is crucial, as is knowing when to call for help. Discussing a "star," an attending said: "I loved having him on call because I knew the patients would get great care."

5. The medical year begins on July 1. Residents and fellows commence their training then, and first-year residents begin as second-year PGYs on that date. Many physicians claim that early July is the most dangerous time to be hospitalized, since one may be cared for by newly hatched trainees.

6. This training program lost its credentials the following year.

7. In medicine, more experienced residents teach less experienced ones and are themselves taught by those who are more advanced in their training. The medical maxim "See one, do one, teach one" is perhaps a bit cynical but also accurate.

8. The attendings kept trying to convince this young doctor to go into intensive care, but when we chatted he quietly made it clear that he wanted a specialty with more money and a less punishing schedule. A charming and intelligent young man, he impressed me as an old-fashioned doctor: His goal was a large

home in a prestigious suburb, a luxury sports car, and an attractive wife who spent her spare time doing volunteer work. He was one of the few young doctors I met during this study who had, or at least openly professed, such retrograde goals. (When I guessed that his wife was beautiful, he assented, and when I ventured that he probably drove a Jaguar, he said no, a Porsche.)

9. Cassell 1991a: 33–59.

10. African American families like this one tend to be extremely distrustful of doctors, especially in a situation like this, where they apparently fear that the doctors will allow their loved one to expire. To me, the resident's suggestion seemed intelligent and compassionate and I wondered whether Minnesota, where Siegfried had practiced, lacked a minority group that was particularly suspicious of doctors, or whether he just did not care about the sensitivities of family members.

11. This is a large plastic needle used to deliver substantial quantities of fluid, or to drain gas or fluid from body cavities. Its size makes insertion somewhat painful without some form of (typically, local) anesthesia.

12. There was a great deal of publicity at the time about New York City police shooting an unarmed African man.

13. Ludmerer 1999: 59.

14. I noticed the same phenomenon when a female attending, who usually worked in the cardiothoracic ICU, was on service in the SICU. A woman leading seemed to give nonverbal permission to female residents to speak their minds.

15. Cassell 1998: 80.

16. This figure comes from the medical year from July 1, 2001, to June 30, 2002. Comparative calculations are problematic, however, since a "tertiary care hospital" such as the Midwest medical center gets the sickest patients, often sent from smaller hospitals who lack the specialists and advanced ICU technology to care for them.

17. There were 556 beds, as opposed to 1,400-odd beds in the Midwest medical center.

18. When the residents teased him, charging that he had a shotgun in back, he responded that Texas law allows a shotgun so long as it is in full view.

Chapter Four

1. In 2000–2001, the Midwest unit had 18 beds, with seven attending physicians taking turns caring for patients. By the summer of 2002, the unit had been enlarged to 24 beds, a move that had been contemplated for some time. Two of the seven attending physicians, both surgeons, no longer worked as intensivists; new trauma surgeons who also worked in the SICU had been recruited. By 2003, the unit had 12 attending physicians; 5 of these did not conduct basic research. As with all ethnographies, I am dealing with a moving target (unlike many ethnographies, however, my being close to the unit makes these changes evident, rather than my leaving the site, so that it becomes somewhat frozen in memory). My descriptions of the unit will concentrate on the time from August 2000 to October 2001, since this is when I spent the most concentrated time conducting fieldwork in the SICU.

2. Anesthesia, internal medicine, surgical critical care, and medical critical care.

3. The indications of this sense of superiority were quiet, and I might have been less sensitive to them had I not been married for 30 years to a physician who taught in a medical school as well as having a private practice. To give just one example, doctors who were trained in a center that outclassed the Midwest center in the prestige hierarchy, frequently referred their time there: "When I was at Mass General. . . ."

4. In 2003, there was more uniformity in the drugs and procedures the attendings administered, if not in their styles of relating to patients and families. A study had been conducted quantifying how various SICU doctors practiced, and protocols were written to standardize many of the drugs ordered by the attending physicians.

5. Pinpoint pupils have several causes, including aggressive administration of opiates (narcotics). Such aggressive administration may be used for pain relief, for anesthesia, or for sedation. Since pinpoint pupils also have other, more sinister, causes (such as an injury to part of the brain called the pons), a drug to reverse any narcotic effect is often administered to help sort out the cause. When I questioned this attending, he admitted that yes, he can smell blood and feces, and he knows things without knowing exactly how he knows them: who will do badly, who needs to be taken to the OR immediately, and so forth. Of course, this is based on evidence, but he cannot quite put his finger on what that evidence is. This is a perfect definition of clinical acumen (for a similar example of knowing something without knowing how one knows it, see Ross 1992: 70–78). Naturally, although clinical acumen can be a potent tool, its predictive accuracy is imperfect.

6. I was told that in subsequent years his rounds took less time; he stopped teaching residents, and they moved more rapidly.

7. This, of course, may be true of many residents and fellows, especially the good ones; they model themselves on respected superiors. This emulation is more evident, however, when they are practicing side by side with those former teachers.

8. Cassell et al. 2003.

9. Frick, Uehlinger, and Zenklusen 2003.

10. Let me note that I am now talking about a relatively small core of devoted nurses, bright, insightful, and knowledgeable about patients, doctors, and hospital activities. Naturally, as much variation among nurses existed as among physicians, and not all were as perceptive, astute, or experienced as this core grouping.

11. In New Zealand, I was fortunate to share an office with a remarkable, intelligent, and knowledgeable nurse in a supervisory position, with whom I could discuss my impressions. My three weeks in Texas were too short to form this kind of relationship with a nurse, although one woman has been extremely helpful answering my subsequent questions by e-mail.

12. With the exception of residents and fellows, where men still outnumber women (although the number of women is increasing), and perhaps lab assistants (where the gender divide is roughly equal).

13. "You're either a bitch or a patsy," said one woman surgeon about the problematic relationships between a highly placed woman and subordinate residents, nurses, and secretaries (Cassell 1998).

14. When questioned about their personal lives, a few of the women surgeons I studied indicated, directly or indirectly, that they had little or no personal life, that the demands of their work had impeded the formation of close and lasting relationships (Cassell 1998). I met no male surgeons in this situation; they all seemed to have found wives willing to put up with their punishing schedules.

15. Murphy and Murphy 1974: 101. Interestingly, a graduate school classmate reported that Murphy believed that the ideal relationship between an anthropologist and his field-assistant-wife was one like his own, where the husband possessed the Ph.D. and academic appointment, while the wife had an M.A., thus, knowing enough to assist him, but not enough to compete. I cannot judge the truth of this assertion.

16. Ibid.: 133–35.

17. Cassell 1991.

18. Phillips 1974.

19. I attended a meeting where the nursing director informed the doctors that she had hired 16 new nurses and that when they finished their orientation, the unit should be up to its full complement of 25 beds. Speaking of the new nurses, she implored the doctors: "Be kind to them, they're babies!"

20. Polanyi 1946: 54.

Chapter Five

1. Buchman et al. 2002.

2. Cassell 1991: 42.

3. 1980; see also 1983a, 1983b.

4. May 1980: 367–68.

5. See Bosk 1979 and Gawande 2002: 47–74.

6. Buchman et al. 2002.

7. See Nuland 1994: 250–53; Brody 1992: chap. 5.

8. I attended a surgical M & M where the case of a 70-year-old man was presented. The patient had three different kinds of cancer with a vascular complication that necessitated the removal of his leg. Although it was medically indicated, the family refused an amputation. He received a vascular procedure and, following the procedure, died in the recovery room. A colleague, known for his willingness to operate on what others considered hopeless cases, wondered whether the procedure should have been performed at all, and the surgeon excused himself by saying, "Well, the family insisted." No one (besides myself) apparently questioned this rationale for performing a dangerous procedure on a mortally ill patient.

9. "Flogging" is a disapproving term used to describe the multiple procedures used to keep a dying patient going. Such procedures prolong their dying, but they offer almost no hope for recovery.

10. The family, who had been alienated from the patient for 25 years, had great difficulty deciding to discontinue care. See the case of Mr. Bascombe, discussed on pages 89–91.

11. This comes from a tape-recorded interview.

12. Bosk 1979.

13. See Buchman et al. 2002: 670–71.

14. The latter speculations come from Dr. Stephen Streat, a New Zealand intensivist.

15. From a tape-recorded interview.

16. Brody 1992.

17. Kollef and Ward 1999.

18. One reason the surgeon gave for refusing to allow the patient to be moved was that the unit was "emotionally invested" in her. This was a patient the intensivists had been trying for some time to transfer. The nurses, amused at the notion of their being "invested" in this woman, reported how the patient had declared to one nurse: "You get the hell out of here, bitch!"

19. Bentham (1789/1823), also phrased as "the greatest good to the greatest number."

20. 1992: 217.

21. See Luce and Rubenfeld 2002; Crippen et al. 2002.

22. 1992: 202.

23. This comes from a tape-recorded interview. A SICU intensivist who read this statement disagreed strongly; he felt the significant statement here was "I may not be ready."

24. 1992: 208.

25. An exception to this were the few families who were connected to a doctor in some way, for whom rules might be bent.

26. Zussman studied two medical intensive care units; I was unable to discover whether they were considered "open," "semi-closed," or "closed," but so far as I could tell, they appeared to be, at least in theory, closed units, with ICU attending physicians having formal responsibility for decision making. Kollef and Ward (1999) report similar findings in a medical ICU.

27. In respect to the difference between paternalistic and maternalistic approaches, he observed: "I don't think that it's a coincidence that in the nursing profession, you know, most are women. And when you get up to the end, and things really get tough emotionally . . . it's the nurses who are the first, typically, to say: 'What are we doing here?' They're the ones who spend most of the day with their patients, seeing their agony, and come to us and say, 'What are we doing here?'"

28. During one such conference with the parents of a dying 23-year-old woman (who had never met with the attending on service the previous week, nor been informed of the seriousness of her condition, until a nurse *insisted* that a fellow tell the parents what was going on), I observed in my fieldnotes: "He told them, but didn't tell him. What I mean is that he used such technical terminology that I'm not sure how much the parents got. He spoke of bleeding from 'multiple sites,' of 'multiple ulcers' (not explaining what ulcers are), of 'profusion,' of 'how she's very hot—40 centigrade, which is 105 Fahrenheit' (without saying this was her temperature). I think he thought he was being very clear, but what he was doing was giving the details, in medical language, rather than saying bluntly, she looks much worse and you'd better be worried. . . . He's a very gentle man and I think its hard for him to call a spade a spade. (He probably thinks he is doing so.)"

29. The permission of the family was obtained before recording was initiated; their permission was again requested at the commencement of each recording.

30. Due to my own mechanical ineptitude, I pressed the wrong button after the family had given permission to be recorded.

31. The patient's husband, who had Power of Attorney, which gave him the authority to make legally binding end-of-life decisions, had finally visited the hospital and discovered that his daughter, who spent most of her time at her mother's bedside, had been concealing her mother's dismal prognosis from him.

32. The attending "signed out" to the next person on service on Sunday afternoon or evening, and the formal rotation began Monday morning.

33. Thus, intensivists spoke of the "manifestations" of "severe irreversible brain damage," of blood pressure medicine "perfusing" the patient's body and brain, of "the clinical situation now," of "medications to support heart function or blood pressure," and of "a matter of time before [the patient] begins to develop failure . . . and possibly need support." Despite the popularity of medical shows such as *ER*, I often wondered how much of this was comprehended by frightened, grief-stricken, medically unsophisticated family members.

34. The Auckland surgeons still visited patients in the ICU and were given a voice, I was told, in whether a patient should be shifted from aggressive to comfort care, although the final decision was made by the intensivists. But then, according to a New Zealand attending physician who spent some time in a surgical training program there, New Zealand surgeons are less macho and martial these days than they were in the past—and as their American counterparts still are.

Chapter Six

1. The patient is given sedatives to decrease awareness of unpleasant stimuli and to diminish anxiety.

2. Most of the Midwest patients were kept at a Ramsay of 3 or 4. The Ramsay score is as follows: (1) anxious and agitated, or restless, or both; (2) cooperative, oriented, and tranquil; (3) responding to commands only; (4) asleep, but responds to physical or auditory stimuli; (5)asleep, but sluggish response to physical or auditory stimuli; (6) no response.

3. Ativan, Fentanyl, and Propofol.

4. I spent a brief time in a Paris medical-surgical ICU, at *l'hopital St. Joseph*, where most patients were also awake; the patient–nurse ratio was also 2 to 1. The New Zealand ICU, on the other hand, had a 1 to 1 nurse–patient ratio.

5. This intensivist also likes to call Propofol "milk of amnesia." An American intensivist disagreed with his remarks, saying that ICU patients who are highly sedated do not have to be flat on their backs: Their beds can be tilted so they do not get pneumonia.

6. Epidural analgesia is a method that relieves pain by feeding local anesthetic continually to the nerve roots as they emerge from the spinal cord within the vertebral (spinal) column; the use of epidural analgesia can reduce or avoid the need for sedatives and narcotic pain relievers. (The technique, however, is not appropriate for all patients and has its own side effects.)

7. Tonelli 1996.

8. It is quite possible that the very realistic fear of lawsuits motivated such behavior, as one intensivist did indeed infer. It may well have been an open secret among the intensivists, never discussed directly with the visiting anthropologist,

that neither the doctors nor the hospital could afford the financial and emotional drain of a lawsuit with an uncertain outcome that might hang over their heads for years before going to court.

9. A tracheotomy, or "trach," is an opening through the front of the neck into the trachea ("windpipe") and insertion of a tube, permitting the attachment of a mechanical ventilator to assist breathing.

10. She would not be cured, but might last longer.

11. *Sepsis* is a term used to refer to the body's response to infection. In the dawn of the antibiotic era, it was hoped that drugs that killed bacteria would function as "magic bullets" and provide miraculous cures. While antibiotics have proved extraordinarily effective in managing infections, many patients remain critically ill and even die, despite appropriate therapy. Modern biology has shown that the infected patient's body becomes a battleground of competing molecules and cells, and that the battle continues long after the cause has been addressed. Such patients are "septic." About 750,000 Americans become septic each year in the United States, and about 500 Americans die each day of sepsis.

12. Attached to the ventilator, which breathes for the patient through a tube inserted into the throat during a tracheotomy.

13. Mr. Bascombe was charged $301,000 for his hospitalization in the ICU, and $42,876 by the surgeons and anesthesiologists who cared for him. Of this, the hospital was reimbursed $98,381 by Medicare. (I was unable to obtain the figures for the doctors' reimbursement, but was told it was probably proportional to the hospital fees.)

14. If indeed he were obstructed, perhaps an operation removing the pancreas, colon, and spleen of a patient with metastatic cancer might be justified as preventing a particularly horrible kind of death. If not, a critic might question the procedure.

15. In another similar case, a 77-year-old woman with diabetes was brought to the Midwest medical center from a nursing home for a vascular operation. At the nursing home, the bedridden patient was unable to turn over without assistance. No blood was reaching her toes, and the family refused the amputation the surgeon recommended, insisting that he attempt to "revascularize" her toes (reconnect the veins so that blood reached her toes). After the operation, the patient "coded" on reaching the SICU and was resuscitated. The daughter, a practical nurse, said she had talked with her mother who had told her that she did not want to live hooked up to tubes. But when a family meeting was held, a distant relative, who was a minister, held forth at length, telling the group it was a sin to allow her to die. Two days later, the daughter decided to shift her mother to comfort care. The cost of the patient's care for this hospitalization added up to $145,682.00. Although Medicare and Medicaid covered much of it, the rest was, as occurs frequently, left unpaid.

16. Mrs. Johnson's fees for her hospitalization were $321,589, of which Medicaid reimbursed $42,292. Her doctors' fees were $42,876 (again, I could not find out whether they were reimbursed, or how much).

17. In asystole, the heart muscles are not contracting at all so there is no heartbeat. (In other arrhythmias found in cardiac arrest, such as ventricular fibrillation, an electric shock across the heart muscle may help individual muscle cells

to synchronize their contractions and give a proper heartbeat.) In asystole, an electric shock will not restore the heartbeat.

18. Nursing home patient Helga Waglie, age 87, was in the hospital in a persistent vegetative state, dependent on the ventilator to breathe. She left no written record of her wishes, and relatives opposed terminating her treatment. The hospital administrators and medical staff took the case to court, where they argued that a physician should not have to provide medical care that does not serve a patient's medical interest. Her husband contended that she would want treatment continued, and in 1991, a Minneapolis probate judge rejected the hospital's position and turned over full guardianship to her 87-year-old husband. The patient died three days later; her medical bill was approximately $750,000.

19. See Blackhall et al. 1999; Degenholz, Meisel, and Lave 2002.

20. European Americans, Korean Americans, and Mexican Americans were also surveyed.

21. Dula 1994: 347.

22. I was conducting research in Texas when this patient came to the SICU.

23. The bills for Mr. Schneider's hospitalization (excluding the fees for the extended care facility) added up to $435,135, of which $150,665 was paid by Medicare and Blue Shield (again, I was unable to determine how much of his $56,775 bills from doctors had been paid). Naturally, although insurance covered much of his care, it may well have been paid for in part by higher rates charged subsequent BlueShield subscribers.

24. 2004: 187.

25. See Wax and Ray 2002 for a discussion of one such case. Such behavior is not necessarily generated by guilt: The newcomer may not have had time to come to terms with loss.

26. 1990: 93.

27. 1988.

28. Jonsen and Toulmin 1990.

29. Many medical ethicists and educators are shifting from a concern with abstract principles to a consideration of stories that illuminate the dilemmas faced by patients and doctors (see Zaner 1993; Charon and Montello 2002).

30. Hunter 1991.

31. Let me note that my "guesstimate" may be off. Mr. Carnegie, despite the intensivists' pessimism, may have had a far better chance of surviving this hospitalization. If these odds do not apply to this particular patient, however, they do apply to many others observed in the SICU, whose surgeons refused to consider shifting them from cure to comfort care.

32. An poignant illustration is provided by surgeon Sherwin Nuland (1994: 252–55), who describes a patient in her 90s whom he persuaded against her will to undergo an operation. "She gave in only to please me," he reports. Afterward, she reproached him for her suffering, and although disturbed, he noted that "the code of the profession of surgery demands that no patient as salvageable as [this woman] be allowed to die if a straightforward operation can save her." He reports that if he had not operated, and allowed the patient to die as she wished, he would have been castigated by his colleagues, at the weekly M & M conference, who would have perceived this death as "a case of poor judgment, if not downright

negligence of the clear duty to save life." Nuland concludes that, "One way or another, the rescue credo of high-tech medicine wins out."

33. 2002.

34. Later, I told her that she had displayed the compassionate behavior I had hoped to observe among women surgeons when I began to study them, which was not as much in evidence as I had anticipated. See Cassell 1998.

35. Casarett, Stocking, and Siegler 1999.

36. He was breathing and still had a corneal reflex, which meant he was not brain dead. But, according to the fellow, he would never recover any consciousness or function.

37. Widespread cancer of the lymph system.

38. The wife had arrived at the hospital carrying several thousand dollars in cash, which she said she and her husband had saved for funeral expenses; a hospital employee took her to the bank to deposit it. When I asked the social worker about her family's refusal to come to the hospital and to help, he said that on occasion, people hoard their money, refusing to help relatives in trouble, who then resent the hoarders and refuse help when necessary.

39. Cassell et al. 2003.

40. One of the surgeons subsequently informed me that the patient had lost 100 additional pounds and was on the way to fulfilling his dream to become "a working productive member of society." He inquired: "If that obese patient had been your 52-year-old brother, would you have pushed to let him go?" From a surgeon's point of view, this patient had "nothing permanent" that doomed him to death, and therefore every effort made to keep him alive was reasonable and utterly justified. I am not sure I would want this surgeon or his colleagues to feel otherwise. The covenantal ethic is vital—for surgeons. And, on occasion, it gets results: patients do recover against all odds. (I return to some of these issues in my discussion of "cheechee" in chapter 10.)

Chapter Seven

1. Dunstan 1985; cited by Crippen 2002: 163.

2. Let me note that these two men were my particular friends, so it is possible I noticed their contributions more than those of their colleagues.

3. After discussing the matter, three of the intensivists summarized the advantages of consensus: "(1) It is good for overall standard and consistency of patient care. It stops the extremes of clinical behavior. (2) It is good for the nurses and the registrars [residents]. They know what to expect and where they stand. They know that things won't change much from day to day or shift to shift. (3) It is good for us. All of us are involved in decisions. It gives us constant peer review. It stops any of us being out on a limb in our clinical practice and gives us medico-legal safety. It helps keep us up to date (it's the discussions about the issues that goes into consensus that does this) and means that none of us fall seriously behind in medical knowledge and advantages. The way we roster [schedule] ourselves with a day about system rather than a week about system helps this too. (4) It gives us great strength in dealing with families, like the ethical dilemmas of patient care. (5) It gives us great strength in dealing with management, other teams

and miscellaneous outside forces (it makes us a formidable opposition). (6) It encourages and supports each others' projects and ideas." Personal communication from James Judson, M.D.

4. How people addressed each other in the Midwest unit varied. Nurses addressed some, but not all, of the intensivists by their first names; everyone addressed nurses and residents by their first names. In the Texas ICU, residents and nurses addressed the doctors as Dr. ____; the intensivists addressed residents and nurses by their first names.

5. The nurses could work 10 12-hour shifts every three weeks, or 5 8-hour shifts weekly; the majority elected the 12-hour shifts.

6. There is a temptation to assign responsibility for keeping patients awake versus "putting them under" to the ratio of nurses to patients. Visiting a medical-surgical ICU in Paris, however (at *l'hopital St. Joseph*), where a staff of 29 nurses on staff and two nurses' aides (plus a nurse-manager and what would be called in the United States a "nurse educator"), alternated working days and nights and weekends to care for 10 patients, I noticed that most of their patients were also awake. In 2001, when I conducted research in New Zealand, on the other hand, there were 66 full-time nurses (or nurse-equivalents) on staff (plus senior nurses) in a 14-bed unit, with 4 additional beds for "high-dependency" patients (there was a 2 to 1 patient–nurse ratio for these patients).

7. An intensivist suggested to a senior nurse that, when the unit had too few patients to keep the nurses busy, rather than giving them unpaid time off, they train the nurses to go to the wards to identify very sick patients who might benefit from the kind of care they give in the ICU.

8. The Midwest medical center had a highly regarded school of nursing, and several ICU nurses were enrolled in their master's degree program; tuition fees were reduced for nurses who worked at the medical center.

9. When a patient is in isolation, they usually have a drug-resistant organism; everyone who goes into the room is supposed to take sterile precautions, such as gloving and gowning, before entering, and then discarding gloves and gowns, so that the organism will not spread to other patients. The SICU had managed to lower their incidence of such organisms by insisting on such precautions. Nevertheless, the fellow ignored them, and superiors ignored his ignoring the precautions.

10. Focus groups our project conducted among family members who had a loved one who had died in the Midwest ICU indicated that most family members thought it was the *nurse* who was in charge of the patient Buchman et al. 2003.

11. The SUPPORT Principal Investigators 1995.

12. The fact that the investigators did not realize they knew nothing about this, and that they would have done well to have had a researcher attached to their project who did, exemplifies the omnipotence and self-assigned omniscience under discussion.

13. I visited another New Zealand unit with an active Bereavement Care Service that brings patients home to die more frequently.

14. The "tearoom" was a feature in the three other New Zealand ICUs I visited, and a doctor who spent time in Ireland told me that Irish units had them as well. This may well be a feature of all British, British-influenced, and formerly

British units. In fact, a book on intensive care in Britain, by a former ICU nurse-sociologist, mentions a 1 to 1 nurse–patient ratio, so that, too, may be a British pattern. Seymour 2001.

15. Fewer critical incidents involving alcohol and violence sent patients to the Auckland ICU. During my 10 weeks of research, one man arrived after being beaten in a bar fight, another was run over by his girlfriend after beating her up, and a woman came to the unit after being beaten by her boyfriend when both were drunk.

16. 2001: 27.

17. Although a new computerized system was in the works, at this stage, the intensivists and residents seemed somewhat dubious about its potential usefulness.

18. The intensivist who described this told me laughingly that the Americans were interested, but they were not satisfied with 95 percent predictability, they wanted a *surefire* way of measuring, ending up with indexes that were so broad that they bring in an unmanageably large number of cases. They wanted no false negatives, he said. This was clearly a New Zealand view of "typical American" overkill.

19. Gammahydroxybuturate. At this time, the drug was freely available on the street and by mail order, ostensibly as a CD cleaner.

Chapter Eight

1. Maori beliefs and practices have permeated New Zealand. Buying a Maori jade pendant, which I had been told one is supposed to receive only as a gift unless it has been blessed to remove the bad luck, I was told by the Pakeha (non-Maori) saleslady that she felt she was "spiritually evolved" enough to bless it for me, before mailing it to the United States. I wondered if she were teasing, but the pendant arrived with a note telling me she had blessed it under a large tree near the crafts shop where I bought it.

2. It is apparently more tolerable in England, and I was told that New Zealand medicine has been influenced by, and is modeled on British medicine. See Payer 1996: 101–23. This will be discussed in more detail in the final chapter.

3. 2001.

4. The government ethical review board stipulated that before I observe end-of-life meetings, a nurse had to obtain permission from family members. We put a notice describing my research on the walls of the little family waiting rooms, and I gave copies to the nurse before she asked permission of families. Only one family refused to have me observe, and this meeting turned out not to deal with end-of-life issues.

5. A PE (pulmonary embolism) is a serious condition where a blood clot (DVT or deep venous thrombosis) that forms in the large veins of the pelvis and legs is carried through the bloodstream and lodges in the pulmonary arteries. When the embolis is large, it can cause sudden and immediate death of the patient. Smaller emboli can cause severe acute heart failure and respiratory failure.

6. CT (computerized tomography) is a type of imaging study that views internal structures. The images are termed "slices," because each image can be thought of as the view one would have if the patient is passed head-to-toe through a

sandwich meat slicer. Here, it was a scan of the pulmonary arteries, which is an excellent test to show (or exclude) the presence of blood clots that have embolized.

7. The one female intensivist was an exception; she wore a dress or a rather elegant suit. When I commented on this, she said that she used to dress less formally, but patients and families used to then take it for granted that she was a nurse, so she shifted to clothing that differentiated her from the scrub-suit clad nurses.

8. CSF drainage, sometimes called EVD (endoventricular drain) consists of a fine catheter passed through the brain into one of the fluid spaces (ventricles) inside the brain to drain the cerebrospinal fluid and reduce pressure buildup. The intensivist felt that because the patient had suffered a severe blow to the back of the head, directly injuring the brain, there was no possibility of survival. The injury to the brain stem had caused it to die; the brain, however, had not yet died.

9. Paget (1998/2004) is one of the few nonmedical writers who emphasize the role of time in medical decisions, and how a correct decision at the moment may seem incorrect in retrospect.

10. This was when potential confounding factors were excluded. The presentation cited Carter and Butt 2001.

11. A member of the Bereavement Follow-up Team contacted the mother. It took seven telephone calls to reach her, and the interview was extremely short, lasting only 10 minutes (the median length of their phone calls is 15 minutes). Despite the fact that this was one of the more experienced nurses on the team, the interview covered no broad subjective content. My informant wondered whether the "closedness" of her responses indicated that the mother was covering up anger or resentment toward the unit or the situation.

Chapter Nine

1. I spent two half-days with the CEO, which is all his crowded schedule would allow.

2. I set up similar rules when I spent a day, or days, following a surgeon, assuring each that it did not hurt my feelings if I were excluded from something that he or she preferred I not observe.

3. In spring 2003, however, this woman left her position at the medical center.

4. These pressures are discussed by Ludmerer (1999: 260–87); among external pressures on academic health centers, he lists the decline of the cities, competition for patients, the new adversarial relationship with government, and "the dawn of the age of limits" as many became more pessimistic about the ability of medical research and care to influence the nation's health, others worried about the rising costs of health care, while the greatest limit was "the lack of vision, leadership and national will to forge a sensible health care policy" (p. 286).

5. The medical center pediatricians, true to their stereotype of being somewhat obedient and childlike, all took the test; administrators had some difficulty, however, compelling the surgeons, who are far more "ornery" and less obedient, to submit to the computer course and exam.

6. A local newspaper reported that the Midwest medical center had disbursed

$350,000 to comply with the new regulations and that an official estimated it would cost approximately $300,000 a year to stay compliant.

7. Ludmerer (1999: 351–52) explains that "the era of cost-containment began in earnest in 1983, when the federal government passed legislation establishing the 'prospective payment' of hospital bills for Medicare patients. . . . Medicare paid a set fee per case, determined by the patient's diagnosis. Diagnoses were placed in one of 467 diagnosis-related groups (DRGs)." If the cost were less than the DRG, the hospital could keep the difference; if the costs ran higher, the hospital would suffer a loss. "Hospitals received a fixed amount of money per case, regardless of their actual expenses." Ludmerer notes that for-profit hospital chains could refuse uninsured patients; most nonprofit community hospitals reduced the amount of charity care they provided. "This left teaching hospitals, together with municipal and veterans hospitals, as the primary dispensers of charity care." "Dumping" began to be practiced, where patients who could not pay would be transferred from private hospitals to teaching or municipal institutions.

8. 2000.

9. Ibid.: 211.

10. Ibid.: 59.

11. Ibid.: 86.

12. The term "compliance" has disturbing connotations, whether used to describe patients following doctors' orders or organizations following federal or JCAHO rulings. It suggests blind obedience to a despotic authority.

13. It must be obvious that I view this "ethical" push for privacy with some skepticism. There are many more significant ethical issues that are not dealt with in hospitals—and the literal-minded "regs" on privacy appear to be an example of trying to catch a butterfly with a Mack truck.

14. Many older nonprofit hospitals have similar center-city locations with similar problems (Cowan 2003: A19).

15. The monthly salary check I received was issued by the School of Medicine.

16. All the chiefs were men, although the heads of some subspecialties were women.

17. 1999: 374.

18. A number of smaller suburban hospitals have done just this, increasing the pressure on the Midwest trauma service.

19. The hospital department of surgery had a militaristic table of organization. At the head was the Surgeon-in-Charge (who also held a medical school appointment as chairman of surgery); this man commanded various "divisions," each with its own chief. General Surgery was one division; it was composed of various "sections," Burn/Trauma/(Surgical) Intensive Care being one of these sections.

20. Let me note that this man was just one of the Midwest medical center surgeons whose "doctor fits" were described to me. No one indulged in a tantrum when I was present, however. I'd like to think I had some magnetic quality that suppressed such scenes, but I suspect this was just the Heisenberg principle in action: The act of observing something affects that which you are observing.

21. Dr. Croci probably perceived, and would consequently describe, the scene quite differently. I observed one incident where a surgeon, upset about what had happened to a patient in the SICU, had a heated conversation with a SICU at-

tending that was subsequently reported as "yelling." It did not sound like yelling to me, nor to a resident listening in, whom I subsequently contacted. Acknowledging the Rashomon Effect means being aware that I am unable to evaluate exactly what went on when I was not present, although "triangulating" several reports from different people, and hearing several tantrums reported for a particular surgeon, does strengthen the impression that someone indulges in "doctor fits."

22. This threat had particular valence since some years earlier, a world-famous surgeon had taken his patients and nurses to the competing hospital; administrators were still working to restore the patient volume and profits formerly brought in by this man's section.

23. When beds were short, the head of trauma, who was also the co-head of the SICU, had the power to cancel operations.

24. When I was studying the New Zealand ICU, an edict came from on high specifying the sum physicians could spend nightly on hotels when they attended meetings (since many of these meetings were in Europe, and the New Zealand dollar had a low exchange rate, these rules were utterly impractical). Another edict limited the amount of horsepower permitted for rented cars.

25. He also observed that if doctors want to find out about working hard they should try pouring concrete for a day (personal communication, James Judson, M.D.).

26. The Auckland intensivists also had the power to cancel operative procedures when they felt there were not enough beds.

27. 1999.

28. Is the difference between the views of these two men, the head of trauma and Eisenberg, due at least in part to the fact that the first man is an administrator as well as a surgeon, and consequently more attuned to the bottom line? Or could it have something to do with surgeons being more hard-nosed than psychiatrists (Eisenberg's specialty)?

29. Blue Ridge Academic Health Group 1998: 11.

30. This report was produced by the Blue Ridge Academic Health Group. This group was founded by the Virginia Health Policy Center at the University of Virginia, and Ernst & Young, who provided "core funding and facilitation." The report is one of a number of Ernst & Young "Publications for the Health Care Industry"; this global firm, specializing in audit, tax, and management consulting, was associated with some organizations, such as Health South and Equitable Life Insurance, subsequently accused of accounting fraud. Ernst & Young was sued by former clients who charged that it had persuaded them to enter into illegal tax shelters; in 2003, the firm was assessed $15 million dollars by the government because it did not properly register tax shelters or maintain lists of people who bought them.

31. A *New York Times* article (Cowan 2003) on the financial difficulties experienced by Mount Sinai Hospital in New York City, notes that consultants have recommended that the hospital press doctors "to be more productive, by seeing more patients or getting more research grants." It quotes a health-policy professor: "'People have been told their salaries will be reduced or their space will be taken away' if they fail to do so."

32. Cluff and Binstock 2001.

33. Steinfels 2001; Kaveny 2001.

34. Kaveny discusses Roman Catholic belief and practice, as opposed to the regime of billable hours, but indicates that other communities might have equally valid approaches to time.

35. Cassell 1991; Katz 1981.

36. Bosk 1979.

37. See Stevens 1971, and Starr 1982.

38. Kaplan, Greenfield, and Ware 1996.

39. Hart and Dieppe 1996: 1606–08.

40. Ludmerer and Fox 2001: 130.

41. Ibid.: 131; Ludmerer 1999.

42. 2001: 216.

43. Weber 1905/2001.

44. 1999.

45. Short and Banthin (1995) estimated that about one-third of the U.S. population younger than 65 years is inadequately insured in any given year. The cutting of the "safety net" and the rising unemployment in 2003 undoubtedly added to the number.

46. 1997.

Chapter Ten

1. 1953: 77.

2. Kass 2002: 226.

3. Payer 1988: 121.

4. Angus, D.C., A. Barnato, W.T. Linde-Zwerble, L.A. Weissfeld, R.S. Watson, T. Rickert, G.D. Rubenfeld. 1994.

5. Personal communication, Jean Carlet, M.D. A similar phrase exists in Italian, personal communication, Massimo Antonelli, M.D.

6. Zussman 1992: 111; Perri Klass tells this story, as well: 1987: 240–41.

7. When the nurse subsequently inquired why he had not used the little room usually devoted to family meetings, he responded: "If I went in there, it would have taken an hour."

8. The ICU team had made various efforts to gradually accustom the patient to breathing on his own without the aid of the ventilator, with no success.

9. In response to my inquiries, I learned that Mr. Bordo was alive two and a half years after the transplant.

10. On successful medical treatment experienced as torture, see Frank 1995: 173–74.

11. Cassell 1991, 1998.

12. Ramsey 1970: 283; quoted in Fox and Swazey 1992: 205.

13. Gawande 2003.

14. Fox 1996.

15. Gawande 2003: 74.

16. Wolfe 1979; Cassell 1991.

17. Bosk 1979; Buchman et al. 2002.

18. Payer 1996: 129.

19. Ibid.: 121.

20. See Dunn 2001; McCahill et al. 2002; Milch and Dunn 2002; Dunn, G.P., R. Milch, A.C. Mosenthal, A.F. Lee, A.M. Esson, J. Huffman 2002; Mosenthal, Lee, and Huffman 2002.

21. Sprung, Cohen, and Sjokvist 1993; Keenan et al. 1997; McLean, Tarshis, Mazer, and Szalai 2000.

22. Carlet et al. 2004; Winter and Cohen 1999; Vincent 1990; Esteban et al. 2001; Ferrand 2001, Prendergast, Claessens, and Luce 1998; Sprung et al. 1993.

23. From Pascal to Bayes to Kolmogorov and the present time, this remains the subtle problem of practical life, including medical practice, where a particular ICU patient will be suffering from several complex disorders in a unique pattern. The findings of epidemiology or evidence-based medicine may provide an array of probabilities, but no refinement of probability theory can provide anything other than generalized guidance. See Faber-Langedoen and Lanken 2000: 887–88.

24. For example, Schneiderman, Jecker, and Jonsen 1990, 1996; Taylor and Lantos 1995; Helft, Siegler, and Lantos 2000; Prendergast 1995.

25. Personal communication, Stephen Streat M.D. Dr. Streat and I discussed these issues when I was in New Zealand in 2002, with further discussion at the 2003 Brussels Consensus Conference. We continued the discussion by e-mail.

26. Personal communication, Stephen Streat.

27. See Cassell, Buchman, Streat, and Stewart 2003.

28. Eleven transplants per million population, compared to 18.6 per million in the United States.

29. See MacIntyre 1981; Putnam 2002. For a discussion of these issues, see Wax 2003.

30. See Levy and Carlet 2001.

31. Carlet et al 2004.

32. See, for example, Curtis and Rubenfeld 2001; Crippen et al. 2002.

33. The Robert Wood Johnson Foundation program on Promoting Excellence in End-of-Life Care (www.promotingexcellence.org). The National Institute of Nursing Research has also funded research in this area, including the project that produced this book.

34. 1991/1925: 160.

35. Another intensivist reported that he discussed these issues with residents during surgical grand rounds.

36. Good and Good 2000.

37. One intensivist with whom I discussed this contradicted my view: "He cares" said the doctor, describing this man sitting at the bedside of a dying patient, holding his hand, "he just doesn't show it." So far as I am concerned, showing it is what caring is about. Nurses reported that he bonded with some families, but paid little attention to others.

38. Buchman et al. 2003.

39. Fox and Swazey 1992: 197–210.

40. Jonas 1993: 158.

41. Levy 2001:31–36.

42. Crippen 2002: 270.

43. For example, Foley 2001; Rubenfeld and Crawford 2001; Luce 2003; Truog 2003.

44. Prendergast and Puntillo 2002; Way, Back, and Curtis 2002; Curtis et al. 2001; Curtis et al. 2002. Also see Lilly, De Meo, Sonna et al. 2000.

45. Abbott, Sago, Breen, Abernethy, and Tulsky 2001; Buchman et al. 2003; Cook 2003.

46. Lilly et al. 2000.

47. Cook 2003.

Appendix

1. Margaret Mead would say this in her classes on anthropological methods.

2. For example, R. Wax 1971; Van Maanen 1988.

3. Mageo 1996; Qureshi 2000.

4. Foster, Scudder, Colson, and Kemper 1979; R. Fernandez 1987.

5. Researchers have described themselves as "halfies" when they had one parent from the group being studied, and another from the Western culture where they received their anthropological training. Abu-Lughod 1991; Narayan 1993.

6. In an anthropology course many years ago, the professor mentioned Paul Radin, who spent so many years among the Winnebago Indians that he felt too much a part of the group to be able to offer an anthropological description and stopped writing about them.

7. Zussman 1992: 235.

8. Ever since the chief of surgery presented me with my first white coat in 1983, I have worn a lab coat when conducting research in hospitals. I do not feel it is deceptive, but it does help me blend into the scenery. In New Zealand, where none of the nurses, residents, or intensivists wore white coats, I wore a nurse's blue scrub suit covered by a flowered top, similar to one worn by some nurses; this had generous pockets for my pen, index cards, and anything else I needed to stow.

9. For example, Zussman 1992: 236; Fox 1959.

10. There have been attempts to make fieldwork more "scientific," with a certain number of pre-planned observations taken in a number of pre-planned sites. In graduate school, I had a young professor trained in this methodology; he had conducted little fieldwork, however, and his research abilities seemed far less impressive than those of my advisor, who apparently just did whatever he felt was necessary in order to learn what he wanted to know.

11. 1979: 193.

12. Cassell 1977, 1991, 1998.

13. Zussman 1992: 234–35).

14. Some fieldworkers keep a separate journal or diary, recording their feelings; in her classes, Margaret Mead said this is how she conducted fieldwork. I find that observations, impressions, and reactions do not need to be separated. See Sanjek (1990) for anthropologists' reflections on fieldnotes.

15. The Ethnograph. Before being introduced to The Ethnograph, I used a similar system, employing 3 × 5 cards containing the codes. The techniques, based

on Glaser and Strauss's "constant comparative method" (1967) were similar, it just took far longer to code, file, and retrieve the notes.

16. Cassell 1978.

17. Geertz 1973.

18. As opposed to an open-ended survey, where the questioner and the person questioned converse, a close-ended survey has room for only brief responses, usually scaled in advance.

19. Anspach 1993: 211.

20. For example, Naroll and Cohen 1970; Pelto and Pelto 1978; Weller and Romney 1990; Bernard 1994.

21. 1974/1855.

22. 1938/1894; 1951/1897.

23. Evans-Pritchard 1964/1951: 71–72

24. 1955/1926: 99.

25. Where he railed about the "niggers" he was studying and made it clear he spent a good deal of time with the expatriate Trobriand community (1967).

26. 1940.

27. For an informed and provocative view of what science is, and is not, see Bauer 1992, who contends that scientists in practice do not actually use what is commonly presented as "the scientific method," and that dispassionate, objective, systematic pursuit of knowledge is more a scientific ideal than actuality; he also argues that those who are most faithful to "the myth" of the scientific method, are social scientists, who (he argues) are not scientists at all.

28. MacIntyre 1981; Putnam 2002.

29. Pickering 1984; Harding 1987; Galison 1987; Smith and Wise 1989; Haraway 1991; Keller 1985, 1992.

30. 1992: 36.

31. Hrdy 1999; Martin 1997a.

32. Kuhn 1970; Lakatos and Feyerabend 1999.

33. Thus, Emily Martin (1997b) points out that the metaphor of the powerful free-ranging sperm finding, penetrating, and fertilizing the passive egg, hence producing the embryo, is more closely related to traditional gender ideology than to what actually occurs when sperm and egg meet.

34. Keller 1985: 7.

35. Cassell 1998.

36. Luhrmann 2000.

37. They have tubes down their throat, making it impossible for them to speak, even if they were sufficiently conscious to do so.

38. See Puri and Weber 1990.

39. The SUPPORT Principal Investigators 1995.

40. Mularski, Bascomb, and Osborn 2001: N21.

41. Curtis et al. 2001; Tulsky, Chesney, and Lo 1995.

42. Field and Cassel 1997: 61–64); Fins and Solomon 2001.

43. E.J. Cassell 1985; Roter and Hall 1992.

44. Cook, Giacomini, Johnson, and Willms 1999; Fins and Solomon 2001; Breen, Abernathy, Abbot, and Tulsky 2001.

45. 1993: 211.

46. Ibid.: 205.

47. Ibid.: 206–8. The Hawthorne Effect refers to a famous series of studies on the productivity of workers where various conditions were manipulated, each change increasing productivity, at least for a time (Mayo 1933); Mayo's conclusions were that being studied increased productivity. (These experiments have subsequently been challenged on various methodological grounds; Kolata 1998). The Heisenberg Effect, also called the Uncertainty or Indeterminancy Principle, specifies that observing something (notably, subatomic particles) alters that which is observed.

48. 1992: 235.

49. Let me emphasize that, despite my embattled tone, I am not criticizing scientific research, not even "scientific" social science research. It is not the only game in town, however, and for certain subjects—those that are emotion-drenched, such as death, and loss, and sorrow—I have doubts that this is the most effective way to proceed. For those who prefer to conduct objective, value-free research, that's fine. Different folks, different strokes. What exasperates me is the tone of superiority so many of these researchers take toward colleagues who seek alternate routes toward understanding. Among the points I'm trying to make is that the definition of "science" (as many feminist critics and philosophers of science have pointed out) is contestable, and that "rigor" is not inevitably yoked to value-free, or soporific, social science.

50. The level of participation does not necessarily divide neatly down disciplinary boundaries: highly participative sociologists and positivist anthropologists exist. To give one example of participation, when sociologist Charles Bosk was conducting research for his outstanding study of surgical training, his interest and enthusiasm so impressed attending surgeons that several offered to sponsor his entry into medical school (1979). Bosk's book, however, was criticized by some social scientific colleagues for its sympathetic portrayal of physicians (personal communication).

51. Cassell 1987.

52. Cassell 1998.

53. In *Rashomon*, a Japanese film produced in 1950, the same event is viewed through the eyes of the four characters who participated. Each view is utterly incompatible with the others, and the film makes no judgment as to what is the "real" truth. The "truth" for each character conflicts with the others' realities.

54. Freidson 1970, 1975; Millman 1978.

55. Medical sociologist Marianne Paget's description of Freidson's writings on medical mistakes as employing "the language of blame and culpability" also applies to Millman's work (Paget 2004/1998: 58–69); Cassell 2002.

56. Jean Briggs's classic dissertation on her life among the Eskimo was one of the earliest of such accounts; it has remained in print since its publication in 1970. I remember hearing a sociologist, who had been an editor at Harvard University Press when the book was accepted for publication, describe the pitched battles as to whether Harvard should publish such a personal, "unscientific" account.

57. Tedlock 1991, 1992.

58. Stoller 1989: 137.

59. Schafer 1992.

60. Charon and Montello 2002; Frank 1995; Jonsen and Toulmin 1990, Zaner 1993.

61. Mattingly 1998; Mattingly and Garro 2000.

62. 1995: 158–63.

63. Fernandez (1991). I have extended Fernandez's evocative phrase to cover narrative as well as metaphorical and metonymic imagery.

References

Abbott, Katherine H., Joni G. Sago, Catherine M. Breen, Amy P. Abernethy, and James A. Tulsky. 2001. "Families Looking Back: One Year after Discussion of Withdrawal or Withholding of Life-Sustaining Support." *Critical Care Medicine* 29(1): 197–201.

Abu-Lughod, Lila. 1991. "Writing Against Culture." In *Recapturing Anthropology: Working in the Present*, edited by Richard C. Fox, 137–62. Santa Fe, NM: School of American Research Press.

Angus, Derek C., Amber Barnato, Walter T. Linde-Zwerble, Lisa A. Weissfeld, R. Scott Watson, Tim Rickert, Gordon D. Rubenfeld, on behalf of the Robert Wood Johnson Foundation ICU End-of-Life Peer Group. 2004. "Use of Intensive Care at the End of Life in the United States: An Epidemiologic Study." *Critical Care Medicine* 32(3): 638–43.

Anspach, Renée R. 1993. *Deciding Who Lives: Fateful Choices in the Intensive-Care Nursery*. Berkeley: University of California Press.

Bateson, Gregory. 1936. *Naven: A Survey of the Problems Suggested by a Composite Picture of the Culture of a New Guinea Tribe Drawn from Three Points of View*. Cambridge: The University Press.

Bauer, Henry H. 1992. *Scientific Literacy and the Myth of the Scientific Method*. Urbana: University of Illinois Press.

Belenky, Mary Field, B. Clinchy, N. Goldberger, and J. Tarule, eds. 1986. *Women's Ways of Knowing: The Development of Self, Voice and Mind*. New York: Basic Books.

Benner, Patricia. 1984. *From Novice to Expert: Excellence and Power in Clinical Nursing Practice*. Menlo Park, CA: Addison-Wesley.

Benner, Patricia, and Judith Wrubel. 1989. *The Primacy of Caring: Stress and Coping in Health and Illness*. Menlo Park, CA: Addison-Wesley.

Bentham, Jeremy. 1823. *Introduction to the Principles of Morals and Legislation*. London: Printed for W. Pickering. (First edition printed in 1780, published in 1789.)

Bernard, H. Russell 1994 *Research Methods in Anthropology: Qualitative and Quantitative Approaches*. Thousand Oaks, CA: Sage.

Blackhall, Leslie, Gelya Frank, Sheila T. Murphy, Vicki Michel, Jocelynne M. Palmer, and Stanley P. Azen. 1999. "Ethnicity and Attitudes Towards Life Sustaining Technology." *Social Science and Medicine* 48: 1779–89.

Blue Ridge Academic Health Group. 1998. *Academic Health Centers: Getting Down to Business.* Cleveland, OH: Health Care Publication Order Department, Ernst & Young.

Bosk, Charles. 1979. *Forgive and Remember: Managing Medical Failure.* Chicago: University of Chicago Press.

Breen, Catherine M., Amy Abernathy, Katherine Abbot, and James A. Tulsky. 2001. "Conflict Associated with Decisions to Limit Life-Sustaining Treatment in Intensive Care Units." *Journal of General Internal Medicine* 16: 283–89.

Briggs, Jean. 1970. *Never in Anger.* Cambridge, MA: Harvard University Press.

Brody, Howard. 1992. *The Healer's Power.* New Haven, CT: Yale University Press.

Buchman, Timothy G., Joan Cassell, Murray L. Wax, and Shawn Ray. 2002. "Who Should Manage the Dying Patient: Rescue, Shame and the Surgical ICU Dilemma." *Journal of the American College of Surgeons* 194(5): 665–73.

Buchman, Timothy G., Shawn Ray, Murray Wax, Joan Cassell, David Rich, Mary Ann Niemczycki. 2003. "Families' Perceptions of Surgical Intensive Care." *Journal of the American College of Surgeons* 196(6): 977–83.

Callahan, Daniel. 1988. *Setting Limits: Medical Goals in an Aging Society.* New York: Touchstone Books.

Carlet, Jean, Lambertus G. Thijs, Massimo Antonelli, Joan Cassell, Peter Cox, Nicholas Hill, Charles Hinds, Jorge Pimentel, Konrad Reinart, and B. Taylor Thompson. 2003. "Statement of the 5th International Consensus Conference in Critical Care, Challenges in End-of-Life Care in the ICU, Brussels, Belgium." 2004. *Critical Care Medicine* 32(5): 2241–45.

Carter, B. G., and W. Butt. 2001. "Review of the Use of Somatosensory Potentials in the Prediction of Outcome after Severe Brain Injury." *Critical Care Medicine* 29(1): 78–86.

Casaret, David, Carol B. Stocking, and Mark Siegler. 1999. "Would Physicians Override a Do-Not-Resuscitate Order when a Cardiac Arrest Is Iatrogenic?" *Journal of General Internal Medicine* 14(1): 35–38.

Cassell, Eric J. 1974. "Dying in a Technological Society. *Hastings Center Studies* 2(2): 31–36.

———. 1976. *The Healer's Art: A New Approach to the Doctor-Patient Relationship.* New York: J. B. Lippincott.

———. 1985. *Talking with Patients: The Theory of Doctor-Patient Communication.* Vol. 1. Cambridge, MA: MIT Press.

Cassell, Joan. 1977. *A Group Called Women: Sisterhood and Symbolism in the Feminist Movement.* New York: David McKay (Longmans).

———. 1978. "Risk and Benefit to Subjects of Fieldwork." *American Sociologist* 13(3): 134–43.

———. 1980. "Ethical Principles for Conducting Fieldwork." *American Anthropologist* 82(1): 28–41.

———. 1981. "Technical and Moral Errors in Medicine and in Fieldwork." *Human Organization* 40(2): 160–68.

———. 1982a. "Harms, Benefits, Wrongs, and Rights in Fieldwork." In *The Ethics of Social Research: Fieldwork, Regulation and Publication,* edited by Joan E. Sieber, 7–31. New York: Springer-Verlag.

————. 1982b. "Does Risk-Benefit Analysis Apply to Moral Evaluation of Social Science?" In *Ethical Issues in Social Science Research*, edited by Tom Beauchamp, Ruth R. Faden, R. Jay Wallace Jr., and Leroy Walters, 144–62. Baltimore: Johns Hopkins University Press.

————, ed. 1987. *Children in the Field: Anthropological Experiences.* Philadelphia: Temple University Press. (Paperback edition 1994.)

————. 1991a. *Expected Miracles: Surgeons at Work.* Philadelphia: Temple University Press.

————. 1991b. "Subtle Manipulation and Deception in Fieldwork: Opportunism Knocks." *International Journal of Moral and Social Studies* 6(3): 269–74.

————. 1998. *The Woman in the Surgeon's Body.* Cambridge, MA: Harvard University Press.

————. 2002. "Social Scientists Studying Doctors." *Reviews in Anthropology* 31(3): 243–62.

Cassell, Joan, Timothy G. Buchman, Stephen Streat, and Ronald M. Stewart. 2003. "Surgeons, Intensivists, and the Covenant of Care: Administrative Models and Values Affecting Care at the End-of-Life." *Critical Care Medicine* 31(5): 1551–59.

Cassell, Joan, and Sue-Ellen Jacobs, eds. 1987. *Handbook of Ethical Issues in Anthropology.* Washington, DC: American Anthropological Association.

Cassell, Joan, and Murray L. Wax, eds. 1980. "Ethical Problems of Fieldwork." *Social Problems* 27(3). (Special issue.)

Chambliss, Daniel F. 1996. *Beyond Caring: Hospitals, Nurses, and the Social Organization of Ethics.* Chicago: University of Chicago Press.

Charon, Rita, and Martha Montello, eds. 2002. *Stories Matter: The Role of Narrative in Medical Ethics.* New York: Routledge.

Chiarella, Mary. 2002. *The Legal and Professional Status of Nursing.* Edinburgh: Churchill Livingstone.

Chodorow, Nancy. 1978. *The Reproduction of Mothering: Psychoanalysis and the Sociology of Gender.* Berkeley: University of California Press.

Cluff, Leighton E., and Robert H. Binstock, eds. 2001. *The Lost Art of Caring: A Challenge to Health Professionals, Families, Communities, and Society.* Baltimore: Johns Hopkins University Press.

Comte, August. 1974. *Cours de Philosphie Positive* [*The Positive Philosophy*] with a New Introduction by Abraham S. Blumberg. Six Vols. New York: AMS Press. (Originally published 1855.)

Connections (newsletter of the Association of Women Surgeons). 2001. (7)2.

————. 2002. 8(1).

Cook, Deborah. 2003. "Optimal Care for Patients Dying in the ICU: Interventions to Improve the Care to Patients Dying in the ICU." Presentation at the International Consensus Conference on Challenges in End-of-Life Care, in Brussels, Belgium, April 2003.

Cook, Deborah, J. Mita Giacomini, Nancy Johnson, and Dennis Willms. 1999. "Life Support in the Intensive Care Unit: A Qualitative Investigation of Technological Purposes." *Canadian Medical Association Journal* 161: 1109–13.

Cowan, Alison. 2003. "How a Venerable Hospital Helped Undermine Its Own Fiscal Health (Mt. Sinai)." *New York Times* April 7: A19.

Crippen, David. 2002. " Afterword." In *Three Patients: International Perspectives on Intensive Care at the End of Life*, edited by David Crippen, Jack K. Kilcullen, and David F. Kelly, 265–70. Boston/Dordrecht/London: Kluwer Academic Publishers.

Crippen, David, Jack K. Kilcullen, and David F. Kelly, eds. 2002. *Three Patients: International Perspectives on Intensive Care at the End of Life*. Boston/Dordrecht/ London: Kluwer Academic Publishers.

Curtis, J. Randall, and Gordon D. Rubenfeld, eds. 2001. *Managing Death in the Intensive Care Unit: The Transition From Cure to Comfort*. New York: Oxford University Press.

Curtis, J. Randall, Donald L. Patrick, Sarah E. Shannon, Patsy D. Treese, Ruth A. Engelberg, Gordon D. Rubenfeld. 2001. "The Family Conference as a Focus to Improve Communication about End-of-Life Care in the Intensive Care Unit: Opportunities for Improvement." *Critical Care Medicine* 29(2): N26–N33.

Curtis, J. Randall, Ruth A. Engelberg, Marjorie D. Wenrich, Elizabeth L. Nielsen, Sarah E. Shannon, Patsy D. Treece, Marck R. Tonelli, Donald L. Patrick, Lynne S. Robins, Barbara B. McGrath, and Gordon D. Rubenfeld. 2002. "Studying Communication about End-of-Life Care during the ICU Family Conference: Development of a Framework." *Journal of Critical Care* 17(3): 147–60.

Daston, Lorraine. 1995. "The Moral Economy of Science." *Osiris* 10: 3–26.

Degenholtz, H. B., Arnold R. Meisel, and J. R. Lave. 2002. "Persistence of Racial Disparaties in Advance Care Documents among Nursing Home Residents." *Journal of the American Geriatrics Society* 50: 378–81.

Devereux, George. 1967. *From Anxiety to Method in the Behavioral Sciences*. New York: Humanities Press.

DiGiacomo, Susan M. 1987. "Biomedicine as a Cultural System: An Anthropologist in the Kingdom of the Sick." In *Encounters with Biomedicine: Case Studies in Medical Anthropology*, edited by Hans A. Baer, 315–46. New York: Gordon and Breach.

Dula, Annette. 1994. "African American Suspicion of the Healthcare System is Justified: What Do We Do about It?" *Cambridge Quarterly of Healthcare Ethics* 3: 347–57.

Dunn, Geoffrey P. 2001. "Patient Assessment in Palliative Care: How to See the 'Big Picture' and What to Do When 'There is No More We Can Do.'" *Journal of the American College of Surgeons* 193(5): 565–73.

Dunn, Geoffrey P. (Moderator), Robert A. Milch, Anne C. Mosenthal, K. Francis Lee, Alexandra M. Easson, and Joan I. Huffman. 2002. "Palliative Care by the Surgeon: How to Do It." *Journal of the American College of Surgeons* 194(4): 509–37.

Dunstan, G. R. 1985. "Hard Questions in Intensive Care: A Moralist Answers Questions Put to Him at a Meeting of the Intensive Care Society, Autumn 1984." *Anaesthesia* 40(5): 479–82.

Durkheim, Emile. 1938. *The Rules of Sociological Method*. Translated by Sarah A. Solovay and John H. Muller, edited by George E. G. Catlin. New York: Free Press. (Originally published 1894.)

———. 1951. *Suicide: A Study in Sociology*. Translated by John A. Spaulding and

George Simpson, edited by Geroge Simpson. New York: Free Press. (Originally published 1897.)

Eisenberg, Leon. 1999. "Whatever Happened to the Faculty on the Way to the Agora?" *Journal of the American Medical Association* 159(19): 2251–56.

Esteban, A., F. Gordo, J. F. Solsona, I. Alia, J. Caballero, C. Bouza, J. Alcala-Zamora, D. J. Cook, J. M. Sanchez, R. Abizanda, G. Miro, M. J. Fernandez Del Cabo, E. de Miguel, J. A. Santos, B. Balerdi. 2002 "Withdrawing and Withholding Life Support in the Intensive Care Unit: A Spanish Prospective Multi-Center Observational Study." *Intensive Care Medicine* 27: 1744–49.

Evans-Pritchard, E. 1940. *The Nuer, a Description of the Modes of Livelihood and Political Institutions of a Nilotic People.* Oxford: Oxford University Press.

———. 1964. *Social Anthropology and Other Essays.* New York: Free Press. (Originally published 1951.)

Faber-Langendoen, Kathy, and Paul N. Lanken. 2000. "Dying Patients in the Intensive Care Unit: Forgoing Treatment, Maintaining Care." *Annals of Internal Medicine* 133: 886–93.

Fernandez, James, ed. 1991. "Introduction." *Beyond Metaphor: The Theory of Tropes in Anthropology.* Stanford, CA: Stanford University Press.

Fernandez, Renate. 1987. "Children and Parents in the Field: Reciprocal Impacts." In *Children in the Field: Anthropological Experiences,* edited by Joan Cassell, 185–215. Philadelphia: Temple University Press.

Ferrand, E., R. Robert, P. Ingrand, F. Lemaire, French Laterea Group. 2001. "Withholding and Withdrawal of Life Support in Intensive Care Units in France: A Prospective Survey." *Lancet* 357: 9–14.

Field, Marilyn, and Christine K. Cassel, eds. 1997. *Approaching Death: Improving Care at the End of Life.* Washington, DC: National Academy Press.

Fins, Joseph J., and Mildred Z. Solomon. 2001. "Communication in Intensive Care Settings: The Challenge of Futility Disputes." *Critical Care Medicine* (supplement): 29: N10–N15.

Fitzgerald, F. Scott. 1991. *The Great Gatsby.* New York: Scribner Paperback Books. (Originally published in 1925.)

Fitzgerald, Maureen. 2001. "Gaining Knowledge of Culture During Professional Education." In *Practice Knowledge and Expertise in the Health Professions,* edited by Joy Higgs and Angie Titchen, 149–56. Oxford: Butterworth Heineman.

Foley, Kathleen. 2001. "Pain and Symptom Control in the Dying ICU Patient." In *Managing Death in the Intensive Care Unit: The Transition From Cure to Comfort,* edited by J. Randall Curtis and Gordon D. Rubenfeld, 103–26. New York: Oxford University Press.

Foster, George M., Thayer Scudder, Elizabeth Colson, and Robert V. Kemper. 1979. *Long-Term Field Research in Social Anthropology.* New York: Academic Press.

Fox, Renée C. 1959. *Experiment Perilous: Physicians and Patients Facing the Unknown.* Glencoe, IL: Free Press.

———. 1996. "Afterthoughts." In *Organ Transplantation: Meanings and Realities,* edited by Stuart J. Youngner, Renée C. Fox, and Laurence J. O'Connell, 252–72. Madison: University of Wisconsin Press.

Fox, Renée C., and Judith Swazey. 1992. *Spare Parts: Organ Replacement in American Society*, 197–210. New York: Oxford University Press.

Frank, Arthur. 1995. *The Wounded Storyteller: Body, Illness, and Ethics*. Chicago: The University of Chicago Press.

Frick, Sonia, Dominick E. Uehlinger, and Regula M. Zuercher Zenklusen. 2003. "Medical Futility: Predicting Outcome of Intensive Care Unit Patients by Nurses and Doctors—A Prospective Comparative Study. *Critical Care Medicine* 31(2): 456–61.

Freidson, Eliot. 1970. *Profession of Medicine: A Study of the Sociology of Applied Knowledge*. New York: Dodd, Mead.

———. 1975. *Doctoring Together: A Study of Professional Social Control*. New York: Elsevier.

Galison, Peter Louis. 1987. *How Experiments End*. Chicago: University of Chicago Press.

Gawande, Atul. 2002. *Complications: A Surgeon's Notes on an Imperfect Science*. New York: Henry Holt and Company.

———. 2003. "Desperate Measures: Francis Moore Remade Modern Surgery. But He Couldn't Live with the Consequences." *New Yorker* May 5: 70–81.

Geertz, Clifford. 1973. *The Interpretation of Cultures*. New York: Basic Books.

Gillet, Grant. 2001. "The RUB." *New Zealand Medical Journal*. April 27: 188–89.

Gilligan, Carol. 1982. *In a Different Voice: Psychological Theory and Women's Development*. Cambridge, MA: Harvard University Press.

Glaser, Barney G., and Anselm L. Strauss. 1967. *The Discovery of Grounded Theory: Strategies for Qualitative Research*. Chicago: Aldine.

Good, Byron J., and Mary-Jo DelVeccio Good. 2000. "'Fiction' and 'Historicity' in Doctors' Stories: Social and Narrative Dimensions of Learning Medicine." In *Narrative and the Cultural Construction of Illness and Healing*, edited by Cheryl Mattingly and Linda C. Garro, 50–69. Berkeley: University of California Press.

Gordon, Deborah R. 1988. "Clinical Science and Clinical Expertise." In *Biomedicine Examined*, edited by M. Lock and D. Gordon, 257–95. Dordrecht: Kluwer Academic Publishers.

Haraway, Donna. 1991. *Simians, Cyborgs, and Women: The Reinvention of Nature*. New York: Routledge.

Harding, Sandra. 1987. "Introduction: Is There a Feminist Method?" and "Conclusions: Epistemological Questions." In *Feminism and Methodology*, edited by Sandra Harding, 1–14, 181–89. Bloomington: University of Indiana Press.

Hart, J. T., and P. Dieppe. 1996. "Caring Effects." *Lancet* 347: 1606–08.

Helft, P. R., M. Siegler, and J. D. Lantos. 2000. "The Rise and Fall of the Futility Movement [comment]." *New England Journal of Medicine* 343(4): 293–96.

Hindwood, B. 1991. "The Nurse in Profile." *The Lamp* 48(8): 48.

Hrdy, Sarah Blaffer. 1999. *Mother Nature: A History of Mothers, Infants, and Natural Selection*. New York: Parthenon Books.

Hunter, Kathryn Montgomery. 1991. *Doctors Stories: The Narrative Structure of Medical Knowledge*. Princeton, NJ: Princeton University Press.

Jonas, Hans. 1993. "The Burden and Blessing of Mortality." In *Bioethics: Basic Writings on the Key Ethical Questions that Surround the Major Modern Biological Possibilities and Problems*, edited by Thomas A. Shannon, 155–66. Mahwah, NJ: Paulist Press.

Jonsen, Alvin R., and Stephen Toulmin. 1990. *The Abuse of Casuistry: A History of Moral Reasoning*. Berkeley: University of California Press.

Kass, Leon R. 2002. "Is There a Right to Die?" In *Life, Liberty and the Defense of Dignity*. San Francisco: Encounter Books.

Katz, Pearl. 1981. "Ritual in the Operating Room." *Ethnology* 20(4): 335–50.

Kaufman, Sharon R. 2001. "Clinical Narratives and Ethical Dilemmas in Geriatrics." In *Bioethics in Social Context*, edited by Barry Hoffmaster, 12–38. Philadelphia: Temple University Press.

Kaveny, M. Kathleen. 2001. "Billable Hours in Ordinary Time: A Theological Critique of the Instrumentalization of Time in Professional Life." *Loyola University Chicago Law Review* 33: 173–220.

Keller, Evelyn Fox. 1985. *Reflections on Gender and Science*. New Haven, CT: Yale University Press.

———. 1992. *Secrets of Life, Secrets of Death: Essays on Language, Gender and Science*. New York: Routledge.

Keenan, S. P., K. D. Busche, L. M. Chen, L. McCarthy, K. J. Inman, and W. J. Sibbald. 1997. "A Retrospective Review of a Large Cohort of Patients Undergoing the Process of Withholding or Withdrawal of Life Support." *Critical Care Medicine* 25: 1324–31.

Kelvin, Baron William Thomson. *Hathaway's stenographic report of twenty lectures delivered in Johns Hopkins University, Baltimore, in October 1884: followed by twelve appendices on allied subjects by Lord Kelvin*. London: C. J. Clay and Sons.

Kolata, Gina. 1998. "Scientific Myths that Are Too Good to Die." *New York Times*. December 6. D 7.

Kollef, M. H., and S. Ward. 1999. "The Influence of Access to a Private Attending Physician on the Withdrawal of Life-Sustaining Therapies in the Intensive Care Unit." *Critical Care Medicine* 27: 2125–32.

Konner, Melvin. 1988. *Becoming a Doctor: A Journey of Initiation in Medical School*. New York: Penguin Books.

Kuhn, Thomas S. 1970. *The Structure of Scientific Revolutions*. Chicago: University of Chicago Press.

Lakatos, Imre, and Paul Feyerabend. 1999. *For and Against Method*. Edited by Matteo Motterlini. Chicago: University of Chicago Press.

Lave, Jean, and Etienne Wenger. 1991. *Situated Learning: Legitimate Peripheral Participation*. Cambridge: Cambridge University Press.

Levy, Mitchell M. 2001. "Making a Personal Relationship with Death." In *Managing Death in the Intensive Care Unit: The Transition From Cure to Comfort*, edited by J. Randall Curtis and Gordon D. Rubenfeld, 31–36. New York: Oxford University Press.

Levy, Mitchell M., and Carlet, Jean, eds. 2001. Compassionate End-of-Life Care in the Intensive Care Unit. *Critical Care Medicine* (supplement) N29(2).

Lilly, C. M., D. L. De Meo, L. A. Sonna, K. J. Haley, A. F. Massaro, R. F.

Wallace, S. Cody. 2000. "An Intensive Communication Intervention for the Critically Ill." *American Journal of Medicine* 109: 469–75.

Lock, Margaret. 2001. "The Tempering of Medical Anthropology: Troubling Natural Categories." *Medical Anthropology Quarterly* 15(4): 478–92.

Luce, John. 2003. "Optimal Care for Patients Dying in the ICU: Withdrawing Life Sustaining Treatments." Presentation at the International Consensus Conference on Challenges in End-of-Life Care, in Brussels, Belgium, April 2003.

Luce, John M., and Mitchell M. Levy, eds. 2001. *Critical Care Medicine* (supplement) 29(2).

Luce, John M., and Gordon D. Rubenfeld. 2002. "Can Health Care Costs be Reduced by Limiting Intensive Care at the End of Life?" *American Journal of Respiratory Critical Care Medicine* 165: 750–54.

Ludmerer, Kenneth M. 1999. *Time to Heal: American Medical Education from the Turn of the Century to the Era of Managed Care.* New York: Oxford University Press.

Ludmerer, Kenneth, and Renée Fox. 2001. "Caring and Medical Education." In *The Lost Art of Caring: A Challenge to Health Professionals, Families, Communities, and Society,* edited by Leighton E. Cluff and Robert H. Binstock, 125–36. Baltimore: Johns Hopkins University Press.

Luhrmann, T. M. 2000. *Of Two Minds: The Growing Disorder in American Psychiatry.* New York: Alfred A. Knopf.

MacIntyre, Alisdair. 1981. *After Virtue: A Study in Moral Theory.* Notre Dame, IN: University of Notre Dame Press.

Mackay, Leslie. 1993. *Conflicts in Care: Medicine and Nursing.* London: Chapman & Hall.

Mageo, Jeanette Marie. 1996. "Spirit Girls and Marines: Possession and Ethnopsychiatry as Historical Discourse in Samoa." *American Ethnologist* 23: 61–82.

Malinowski, Bronislaw. 1955. "Myth in Primitive Psychology." In *Magic, Science and Religion and Other Essays,* 93–148. New York: Doubleday Anchor. (Originally published 1926.)

———. 1967. *A Diary in the Strict Sense of the Term,* translated by Norbert Guterman. New York: Harcourt, Brace & World.

Martin, Emily. 1997a. "How Science Has Constructed a Romance Based on Stereotypical Female-Female Roles." In *Situated Lives: Gender and Culture in Everyday Life,* edited by Louise Lamphere, Helena Ragoné, and Patricia Zavella, 85–98. New York: Routledge.

———. 1997b. "Medical Metaphors of Women's Bodies: Menstruation and Menopause." In *Writing on the Body: Female Embodiment and Feminist Theory,* edited by Katie Conboy, Nadia Medina, and Sarah Stanbury, 15–41. New York: Columbia University Press.

Mattingly, Cheryl. 1998. *Healing Dramas and Clinical Plots: The Narrative Structure of Experience.* Cambridge: Cambridge University Press.

Mattingly, Cheryl, and Linda Garro, eds. 2000. *Narrative and the Cultural Construction of Illness and Healing.* Berkeley: University of California Press.

May, William F. 1980. "Doing Ethics: The Bearing of Ethical Theories on Fieldwork." *Social Problems* 27:3 (special issue on Ethical Problems of Fieldwork, edited by Joan Cassell and Murray W. Wax): 358–70.

————. 1983a. *The Physician's Covenant: Images of the Healer in Medical Ethics.* Philadelphia: Westminister Press.

————. 1983b. *Testing the Medical Covenant: Active Euthanasia and Health Care Reform.* Grand Rapids, MI: William B. Eerdmans.

Mayo, Elton. 1933. *Human Problems of an Industrial Civilization.* New York: Macmillan.

McCahill, Laurence E., Robert S. Krouse, David Z. J. Chu, Gloria Juarez, Gwen C. Uman, Betty R. Ferrell, and Lawrence D. Wagman. 2002. "Decision Making in Palliative Surgery." *Journal of the American College of Surgeons* 195(3): 411–22.

McLean R. F., J. Tarshis, C. D. Mazer, and J. P. Szalai. 2000. "Death in Two Canadian Intensive Care Units. Institutional Differences and Changes over Time." *Critical Care Medicine* 28: 100–103.

Milch, Robert A., and Geoffrey P. Dunn. 2002. "Communication: Part of the Surgical Armamentarium." *Journal of the American College of Surgeons* 193(4): 449–51.

Millman, Marcia. 1978. *The Unkindest Cut: Life in the Backrooms of Medicine.* New York: Morrow.

Mosenthal, Anne C., K. Francis Lee, and Joan Huffman. 2002. "Palliative Care in the Surgical Intensive Care Unit." *Journal of the American College of Surgeons* 194(1): 75–83.

Mularski, Richard, Paul Bascomb, and Molly L. Osborn. 2001. "Educational Agendas for Interdisciplinary End-of-Life Curricula." *Critical Care Medicine* (supplement) 29: N16–N23.

Murphy, Yolanda, and Robert F. Murphy. 1974. *Women of the Forest.* New York: Columbia University Press.

Narayan, Kirin. 1993. "How Native is a 'Native' Anthropologist?" *American Anthropologist* 95(3): 671–85.

Naroll, Raoul, and Ronald Cohen, eds. 1970. *A Handbook of Methods in Cultural Anthropology.* Garden City, NY: Natural History Press.

Noddings, Nell. 1984. *Caring: A Feminine Approach to Ethics and Moral Education.* Berkeley: University of California Press.

Nolen, William. 1950. *The Making of a Surgeon.* New York: Random House.

Nuland, Sherwin B. 1994. *How We Die: Reflections on Life's Final Chapter.* New York: Alfred A Knopf.

Osler, William. c.1900. "Nurse and Patient." Reprinted in 1987. *Aequanimitas, with Other Addresses to Medical Students, Nurses, and Practitioners of Medicine,* 163. Birmingham, AL.: Classics of Medicine Library.

Paget, Marianne A. 2004. *The Unity of Mistakes: A Phenomenological Interpretation of Medical Work.* Philadelphia: Temple University Press. (Originally published in 1988.)

Payer, Lynn. 1996. *Medicine and Culture: Varieties of Treatment in the United States, England, West Germany, and France.* New York: Henry Holt and Company.

Pelto, Perti J., and Gretel H. Pelto. 1978. *Anthropological Research: The Structure of Inquiry,* 2nd ed. Cambridge: Cambridge University Press.

Phillips, Susan U. 1974. "Warm Springs 'Indian Time:' How the Regulation of Participation Affects the Progression of Events." In *Explorations in the Ethnog-*

raphy of Speaking, edited by Richard Bauman and Joel Sherzer, 92–109. New York: Cambridge University Press.

Pickering, Andrew. 1984. *Constructing Quarks: A Sociological History of Particle Physics*. Chicago: University of Chicago Press.

Polanyi, Michael. 1946. *Science, Faith and Society*. Chicago: University of Chicago Press.

Prendergast, T. J. 1995. "Futility and the Common Cold: How Requests for Common Antibiotics Can Illuminate Care at the End of Life." *Chest* 107(3): 836–44.

Prendergast, T. J., M. T. Claessens, and J. M. Luce. 1998. "A National Survey of End-of-Life Care for Critically Ill Patients." *American Journal of Respiratory Critical Care Medicine* 158: 1163–67.

Prendergast, Thomas J. and Kathleen A. Puntillo. 2002. "Withdrawal of Life Support: Intensive Caring at the End of Life." *Journal of the American Medical Association* 288(21): 2732–40.

Puri, Vinod K., and Leonard J. Weber. 1990. "Limiting the Role of the Family in Discontinuation of Life-Sustaining Treatments." *Journal of Medical Humanities* 11(2): 91–98.

Putnam, Hilary. 2002. *The Collapse of the Fact/Value Dichotomy and Other Essays*. Cambridge, MA: Harvard University Press.

Qureshi, Regula. 2000. "How Does Music Mean?" *American Ethnologist* 27: 805–38.

Ramsey, Paul. 1970. *The Patient as Person: Explorations in Medical Ethics*. New Haven, CT: Yale University Press.

Redfield, Robert. 1953. *The Primitive World and Its Transformations*. Ithaca, NY: Cornell University Press.

———. 1955. *The Little Community*. Chicago: University of Chicago Press.

Reinhardt, Ewe E. 1997. "Wanted: A Clearly Articulated Social Ethic for American Health Care." *Journal of the American Medical Association* 278(17): 1446–47.

Ross, Rupert. 1992. *Dancing with a Ghost: Exploring Indian Reality*. Ontario, CA: Octopus Publishing Group.

Roter, Debra L., and Judith A. Hall. 1992. *Doctors Talking with Patients, Patients Talking with Doctors: Improving Communication in Medical Visits*. Westport, CT: Auburn House.

Rubenfeld, J. Gordon, and Stephen W. Crawford. 2001. "Principles and Practice of Withdrawing Life-Sustaining Treatment in the ICU." In *Managing Death in the Intensive Care Unit: The Transition from Cure to Comfort*, edited by J. Randall Curtis and Gordon D. Rubenfeld, 127–48. New York: Oxford University Press.

Sanjek, Roger, ed. 1990. *Fieldnotes: The Makings of Anthropology*. Ithaca, NY: Cornell University Press.

Sargant, William. 1957. *Battle for the Mind: A Physiology of Conversion and Brain-Washing*. London: Wm. Heineman, Ltd.

Schafer, Roy. 1992. *Retelling a Life: Narration and Dialogue in Psychoanalysis*. New York: Basic Books.

Schneiderman, L. J., N. S. Jecker, and A. R. Jonsen. 1990. "Medical Futility: Its Meaning and Ethical Implications." *Annals of Internal Medicine* 112: 949–54.

———. 1996. "Response to Critiques." *Annals of Internal Medicine* 125: 669–74.

Seymour, Jane E. 2001. *Critical Moments—Death and Dying in Intensive Care.* Buckingham, UK: Open University Press.

Shaw, Alison. 2003. "Interpreting Images: Diagnostic Skill in the Genetics Clinic." *Journal of the Royal Anthropological Institute* 9(1): 39–53.

Shepherd, Naomi. 1993. *A Price Below Rubies: Jewish Women as Rebels and Radicals.* Cambridge, MA: Harvard University Press.

Short, Pamela Farley, and Jessica S. Banthin. 1995. "New Estimates of the Underinsured Younger than 65 Years." *Journal of the American Medical Association* 274(16): 1302–06.

Silvester, Edward J. 2004. *Back from the Brink: How Crises Spur Doctors to New Discoveries about the Brain.* Washington, DC: Dana Press.

Smith, Crosbie, and M. Norton Wise. 1989. *Energy and Empire: A Biographical Study of Lord Kelvin.* Cambridge: Cambridge University Press.

Sontag, Susan. 1978. *Illness as Metaphor.* New York: Farrar, Straus and Giroux.

Sprung, C. L., H. H. Bulow, S. Hovilehto, D. Ledoux, A. Lippert, P. Maiai, D. Phelan, W. Schobersberger, E. Wenberg, T. Woodcock, ETHICUS Study Group. 2003. "End of Life Practices in European Intensive Care Units—The ETHICUS Study." *Journal of the American Medical Association.* 290(6): 790–97.

Starr, Paul. 1982. *The Social Transformation of American Medicine.* New York: Basic Books.

Steinfels, Peter. 2001. "How Should Time be Lived? A Professor Sees a Billable Hours Culture and Religious Antidotes." *New York Times.* December 29: A10.

Stevens, Rosemary. 1971. *American Medicine and the Public Interest.* New Haven, CT: Yale University Press.

Stoller, Paul. 1989. *The Taste of Ethnographic Things: The Senses in Anthropology.* Philadelphia: University of Pennsylvania Press.

The SUPPORT Principal Investigators. 1995. "A Controlled Trial to Improve Care for Seriously Ill Hospitalized Patients: The Study to Understand Prognoses and Preferences for Outcomes and Risks of Treatments (SUPPORT)." *Journal of the American Medical Association* 274(20): 1591–98.

Taylor, R. M., and J. D. Lantos. 1995. "The Politics of Medical Futility." *Issues in Law & Medicine* 11(1): 3–12.

Tedlock, Barbara. 1991. "From Participant Observation to the Observation of Participation: The Emergence of Narrative Ethnography." *Journal of Anthropological Research* 47: 69–94.

———. 1992 *The Beautiful and the Dangerous: Encounters with Zuni Indians.* New York: Penguin.

Thernstrom, Melanie. 1994. "The Writing Cure: Can Understanding Narrative Make You a Better Doctor?" *New York Times Magazine Section* April 18: 42–47.

Thomas, Dylan. 1953. "And Death Shall Have No Dominion." "Do Not Go Gentle Into that Good Night." In *The Collected Poems of Dylan Thomas 1934–1953.* New York: New Directions Books, 77, 128.

Thomas, William Issac. 1966. *W. I. Thomas on Social Organization and Social Personality: Selected Papers,* edited and with an introduction by Morris Janowitz. Chicago: University of Chicago Press.

Thompson, E. P. 1991. *Customs in Common London.* London: Merlin Press.

Tonelli, Mark R. 1996. "Pulling the Plug on Living Wills: A Critical Analysis of Advance Directives." *Chest* 110: 816–22.

Truog, Robert. 2003. "Optimal Care for Patients Dying in the ICU: Sedation, Pain Control and Paralysis." Presentation at the International Consensus Conference on Challenges in End-of-Life Care, in Brussels, Belgium, April 2003.

Turner, Victor. 1967. "Betwixt and Between: The Liminal Period in *Rites de Passage.*" In *The Forest of Symbols: Aspects of Ndembu Ritual,* 93–111. Ithaca, NY and London: Cornell University Press.

van Gennep, Arnold. 1960. *The Rites of Passage,* translated by Monika B. Vizedom and Gabrielle L. Caffee. Chicago: The University of Chicago Press.

Van Maanen, John. 1988. *Tales of the Field: On Writing Ethnography.* Chicago: University of Chicago Press.

Vincent, J. L. 1990. "European Attitudes Toward Ethical Problems in Intensive Care Medicine: Results of an Ethical Questionnaire." *Intensive Care Medicine* 16: 256–64.

Wax, Murray L. 2003. "Creating Compassionate Care within the Hospital Intensive Care Unit: Beyond Positivism and Toward Wisdom and Responsibility." *Qualitative Research* 3(1): 119–38.

Wax, Murray L., and Joan Cassell, eds. 1979. *Federal Regulations: Ethical Issues and Social Research.* Boulder, CO: Westview Press, for the American Association for the Advancement of Science.

Wax, Murray L., and Shawn Ray. 2002. "Dilemmas within the Surgical Intensive Care Unit." *Journal of the American College of Surgeons* 195(5): 721–28.

Wax, Rosalie H. 1971. *Doing Fieldwork: Warnings and Advice.* Chicago: University of Chicago Press.

Way, Jenny, Anthony Back, and J. Randall Curtis. 2002. "Withdrawing Life Support and Resolution of Conflict with Families." *British Medical Journal* 325: 134–35.

Weber, Max. 1946 *From Max Weber: Essays in Sociology,* edited and translated by H. H. Gerth and C. Wright Mills. New York: Oxford University Press.

———. 1968. *Wirtschaft und Gesellschaft,* edited and translated by Guenther Ross and Claus Wittich. New York: Bedminister. (Originally published 1921.)

———. 2002. *The Protestant Ethic and the "Spirit" of Capitalism and other Writings,* edited and translated by Peter Baehr and Gordon C. Wells. New York, London: Penguin Books. (Originally published 1905.)

Weller, Susan, and A. Kimball Romney. 1990. *Metric Scaling: Correspondence Analysis.* Newbury Park, CA: Sage.

Wiener, Carolyn L. 2000. *The Elusive Quest: Accountability in Hospitals.* New York: Aldine De Gruyter.

Winter, B., and S. Cohen. 1999. "ABC of Intensive Care. Withdrawal of Treatment." *British Medical Journal* 319: 306–08.

Wolfe, Tom. 1979. *The Right Stuff.* New York: Random House.

———. 1987. *Radical Chic and Mau-Mauing the Flak Catchers.* New York: Farrar, Straus and Giroux. (Originally published 1970.)

Zaner, Richard M. 1993. *Troubled Voices: Stories of Ethics and Illness.* Cleveland: Pilgrim Press.

Zussman, Robert. 1992. *Intensive Care: Medical Ethics and the Medical Profession.* Chicago: University of Chicago Press.

Index

Joan Cassell is a Research Associate in the Department of Surgery at the Washington University School of Medicine. She is the author of *Expected Miracles: Surgeons at Work* (Temple) as well as *A Group Called Women: Sisterhood and Symbolism in the Feminist Movement*; *Children in the Field: Anthropological Experiences* (Temple); and, most recently, *The Woman in the Surgeon's Body*.